DEFYING GOLIATH

Settling the Conflict Within

David Michael Como Jr.

www.Defyinggoliath.com
NEW HEIGHTS PUBLISHING

DEFYING GOLIATH
Settling the Conflict Within
by David Michael Como Jr.

Copyright 2008
All Rights Reserved
Printed in the United States of America

ISBN: 978-0-9819115-0-2

The author suggests that all advice given be taken in with a great deal of thought and reason. It is the author's opinion that each individual has a certain responsibility to realize that we are all accountable for our own lives, and must act in accordance with that rule of thumb. The reader should also understand that this has been the author's personal experience, and opinions may vary, simply due to the nature of the subject. The fact is, life holds no absolutes; if this is what is being searched for, than the message of the author has already been compromised.

To my mother and Charlene, two women who helped shape my life into manhood. My mother was the first to show me the strength of a woman's will and determination. She portrayed so well the meaning of unconditional love. Charlene was a remarkable woman who made me realize God.

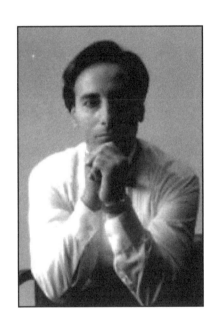

ACKNOWLEDGMENTS

I am so grateful to a dedicated profession devoted to easing the ills of society. The last twenty-seven years of close relations with physicians and nurses have left me with respect and appreciation for their services. From my experience, I have found medicine to be a selfless profession. As thoughts of the past resurfaced in my writing, there was never a moment that I did not reflect endearingly upon the beautiful people tending to me by my bedside. I still remember most of the relationships, even as far back as the day I was first admitted into the hospital. That is the impression they have made on me.

By spending so much time in the hospital through the years I had a front row seat to some of the best of humanity at work. I saw acts of compassion. I was able to witness stunning procedures performed with precision and without hesitation. This left me in awe.

I learned many ways of social interaction just by the way these medical professionals related to me. I knew that that was the way people should communicate, that was the way we should all treat each other—with care and dignity.

Here I am so many years later, and I haven't lost faith in them—not at all. I still believe in what they can do in a crisis.

While self-maturation has not changed in any way what they've been to me, what they've been to me has indeed helped mature me.

I will never be able to repay all those who assisted in my recovery through the years, or acknowledge each individual personally, but I can offer my sincere gratitude for being there when I needed them. Their support will never be forgotten.

Finally, I would like to mention a man who came on board toward the end, when I needed someone's expertise, insight and honest objectiveness. I was not disappointed. James Abraham, my editor and now my friend, was that person. In order for this book to soar to new heights, it must first possess the essentials for flight; he saw to this.

Thank you and God bless you all.

David Michael Como Jr.

PREFACE

When they send you home to "get your affairs in order," saying, in effect, that they've done everything they could, that's the time to shift the gears in overdrive. That is the time to rebel.

No one should tell you what the future will hold for you. No one should have that kind of sway over another, or be allowed to for that matter. That is not a true freedom.

Freedom is forging our own destiny with no submissiveness, creating something from nothing; that's what life does. And what is life? Life flows through us with an unyielding force capable of the most remarkable possibilities, and we are part of it.

I can still hear my mother as clearly today as five or even ten years ago, pleading with me to, "Hurry and get this book out or it will be too late. You will have missed your time!"

I understood her concern and she would've been right if what I had to share was a flavor of the day. Something inside me knew that what I was in touch with had much more to do with human spirit than human interest, which, in my experience, wavers with the wind.

This story embraces that desire to let in the beauty life shows us so often, but most subtly. It is a story about taking chances when it seems safer not to. More than my own biography, it's a story about finding ourselves when all is thought to be lost, in the midst of all despair. It's a story about stepping away from the rat race of society in order to heal both inwardly and outwardly in the only manner appropriate for a complete recuperation.

I intend to explain how miracles are within reach of us all. I separate some of life's distractions from what is most important, and declare some of life's gifts of promise and hope, revealing hints of a living a mystery which has the potential to heal deeply, thoroughly and most convincingly.

Keep in mind that change is most often resisted and sometimes feared, but be assured that life always changes. Life is in constant motion, either pushing silently unnoticed, ever gently in an ebb and flow, or thrusting violently forward with the greatest force imaginable.

Life impresses on us whether we like it or not. It is, however, our response to this influence—or more, our involvement—which matters most. We must find a way to engage in this mystery if we are to benefit from its healing ways.

Though I keep hearing how most people are prone to weakness and lack patience, I see things differently; to me, we're just not completely convinced. We've been caught up in hype, quick solutions, and a dull sense of vagueness. In many ways this can be discouraging.

I love the people around me; I see their beauty, strength and innocence where others do not. I also see a new way ahead, a vision of independence *and* interdependence; both are necessities of life.

This is why I need you with me for more reasons than I have space to write. I have been alone through much tribulation and have somehow learned a way to escape the terrible effects of loneliness, but I would much rather be with family, friends and strangers. I have been blessed with the kind of passion that does not dissipate in time. In fact, it has actually intensified the more that I matured. The closer I get to truth the more I feel and want to share what I know about this wonderful healing mystery. The momentum is already underway and it is undeniable to me. It is individually and secretly capturing the hearts and minds of those rebel-young, as it has mine, no matter what one's age.

I invite all who are interested in living boundlessly in mind to join me as we forge a new way from the old. Through this, together, we will live through cancer and see a day when this threat is no more.

— *Author*

TABLE OF CONTENTS

DEFYING GOLIATH

LIVIN' THE HARD WAY

*There are times when
the only way forward is through the past.*

I was very young when the unnerving thought of death crept into my mind. There it would remain while I gave it a presence it did not or should not ever deserve.

We were three young boys huddled just outside our mother's bedroom—terrified—knees shaking, as our little Beatles cropped heads weaved and bobbed in and out, up and down, to see past the big firemen and gear-toting paramedics, standing over and tightly gathered around our reason for life, who lay there—still—on her bed. We were the quietest we'd ever been in our short time on earth—and that was saying something.

Louie and I tucked Tommy between us as we watched and listened for any hope that mom would get up of her own doing. I looked down to see Tommy in tears. He couldn't have been more than five or six years old. I was about ten and Louis had a year and a half on me.

A stretcher soon whisked by us as our father, unable to hold concern from his eyes, gently grabbed our shoulders and led us into another room. Our mother was carried out the door and into the ambulance, its flashing red lights subdued by the midday sun.

Each one of us took away our own torment from that moment. Either it was shoved deep down and away like our dirty clothes, hidden haphazardly underneath our beds, or it was chased away the moment we found out our mother would be all right. For me, unfortunately, it was the former.

Like a long cast shadow from that very instant in time, fear followed me. It would be many years before I learned that fear has a way of surfacing from these emotional depths no matter how much you turn from it or try to repress it. The truth was, seeing my mother in such a way devastated me.

I felt deeply about life and those I loved. When coming across the unfamiliar, it would be just like me—curious enough to look into things more closely—to leave virtually no stone unturned, even if this meant inviting danger. I sought to make some sense of what I couldn't easily explain away. When those around me feared what could not be understood, it bothered me. I wasn't comfortable with such dreadful mysteries others seemed to settle with so readily.

As I look back to those times, I realize that I had absorbed more from the outside world than I was prepared for at my age. What had happened to my mother made me see that life was strangely unpredictable, and easily could turn my world upside down within a moment's notice.

However, that time life was forgiving. The danger eventually did pass, and time distanced us all from that day. Our mother came home to us. But this new knowledge didn't sit well with me; instead it simmered there on the back burner of my mind, where I slowly gave it strength through the years. It's unfortunate that I was exposed to things of this serious nature while so young, but I think what really made the difference was that I took life for its word. I wasn't one to overlook intention, so when it came to me, I didn't forget. Time could not so easily shut that door for me; my emotions were wedged in between.

I heard about cancer early on in my life. It had slipped out off the tongues of my elders who didn't realize that I was paying attention. I had seen how catastrophic cancer's effect could be, thus I related it intimately with dying. I could not escape the realization that something out there was able to indiscriminately pluck precious loved ones from their families. We were all more or less powerless to do anything about it.

Cancer to me at that time, with what little I knew, was violent, brutal, indecent, shameless and cowardly. It was a senseless, destructive force, lacking meaning or purpose, trespassing into lives without so much as hi or goodbye. This alone was able to put the fear of God in me—very early on. I remember even trying to negotiate with God so that he would spare the ones I loved.

I had religion to protect me in some way, but I wasn't to know for some time that even this would not be enough to calm me. It just didn't make sense to me—feeling so desperate for peace, while enveloped by scripture and congregation. I did what anyone would do when there was the slightest doubt, I held tighter to my beliefs. I wrapped them around me like a heavy warm blanket.

I can see myself walking to church on a Saturday evening, alone, where I would perch in the closest pew to the altar, no more than eleven or twelve years old, wondering what brought me there, yet not wanting to leave.

It was a time when most seats were empty. The many windows of stained glass that would normally allow the brilliant sun to cast light upon the altar and reflect stains of lavender, ruby, jade and gold, against the great wooden pillars that arch together at center—on a Sunday morning—were instead shadowed by the night. I was not inspired by this like so many who gathered once a week in daylight to replenish their spiritual reserves. I was there for another reason, a much darker reason, and the nocturnal sky reflected this mood. The night intensified my feelings of fear, which is probably why I sought comfort in the church at that hour.

Something had a hold of my spirit and it wouldn't let go, no matter what rituals of prayer I performed or how much dedication I showed by attending mass.

In spite of this, I would find a way to go on, and surprisingly even thrive, without anyone knowing my deepest fears. I managed this heavy load the best way I could.

I found refuge in sports. It did more for me to take my mind away from this feeling than anything else could ever have. It was the balance that kept me level through the years. Nothing felt better or more liberating to me than to push my body, and unconsciously, my will as well, as far as it could go.

My older brother and I were always athletic. We had our father to thank for this. He was the first one to involve us in football, hockey and baseball. After work he would set up the garage with opposing goals and we would play until supper time, and on many occasions well after.

He would be the quarterback in the street, drawing plays on the palm of his hand, as my brother and I ran back and forth about a hundred times between two telephone poles. We enjoyed every minute of it and also the attention our father was giving to us. Whether for organized sports, or just playing in our garage, our father always gave us the best equipment money could buy. We were never without.

In the neighborhood, we played more primitive games which sent us running through yards while getting yelled at. We hid behind bushes, trees, or anything that would conceal us from the other kids. We played whiffle ball down the road, by the boulder at Billy's house, and Nerf football between the same two telephone poles. We would have to be dragged in the house before we'd quit. It was only our father's all-too-familiar whistle which sent us scurrying for the door, well after the street lights had lit up the night; our cheeks flushed crimson with the greatest life force.

I lived with vitality and doom side by side, ever close to my spirit; one thrust me into daring adventure, while the other lingered silently, smothering any hope of lasting confidence. Every now and then I was reminded that all this could be taken away from me at any time. I really don't know why I kept entertaining these fearful thoughts of dying or losing someone I loved. They were just there—right in front of me, and I was too inexperienced to reason them away. The mind can be a loaded gun if not respected, managed and understood.

There was however, another side of me up and coming but not yet realized; a part of me that rebelled from when I was very little. Of course it was my mother who first saw the devil's mischief dashing through my eyes—right from the start. But I'm pretty certain everyone knew it by the time I was just old enough to find trouble. There was little doubt in anyone's mind of my rebellious nature. This reflected an inherent craving to know pure truth, truth without interpretation.

I remember looking around for the tallest trees that I could find. It didn't matter in whose yard they stood; I would climb them anyway, just to reach the top. Huge maples were my favorite, but any old tree would do. When I found one to my liking, I would shimmy and grapple all the way up until the tip started to sway. From there I could see the distant horizon as I wondered beyond—but not nearly long enough.

When my friends tagged along, they would dare themselves half way up the tree, risking no more, looking up—scared for me, yet in awe. I found some separation in this, but only briefly, and not enough to understand what set me apart from some.

My mother would often get a call as I was climbing down from some frantic neighbor worried about me falling out of their tree. But I was long gone before anyone could find me. This was how I lived. This was how I managed to get by in an 'unfair' world. In this manner, death was 'just' if I fell, because I knew what I was up against, as much as I could understand at that age anyhow. The threat was right in front of me, with no shades of gray.

But thoughts of dying at the hand of disease scared the hell out of me. I didn't like the idea of this silent destroyer—cancer—so close to me in thought. It didn't play fair; there was no justice in its actions.

And still, there was the religion that I knew. It did what it could to make sense of the unknown, calm our natural fears, and provide somewhat of a direction for its followers. It was brought into my world from the moment I opened my eyes for the first time, in that I was baptized Catholic. So I looked to this particular tradition for inspiration and strength. I think this is where the true conflict within me began. There might have been a latent rebellion brewing within me that I hadn't been conscious of at that time, but the tension certainly was mounting. To be aware of dying while so impressionable and without proper guidance left me in the grips of the very thing that I feared and empowered for so long. My untamed fear was the means for it to find me, leaving me vulnerable well before I could see this encounter with death as it hurled itself directly toward me.

So the stage was set for its inevitable approach. And while no trumpets blared to warn me of this impending threat to come, indeed it came for me one fateful day…on its chariot, trampling thunderously on my freedom, without fear or favor, manner or mercy.

A little more than twenty-seven years has spent itself against the backdrop of time since that early, brisk, November morning. It was the day that life as I knew it would abruptly end. It followed my last verdant summer, the summer that dramatically changed the course I was on. It was a time when I had squandered my first love and also lost my best friend—forever.

Sometimes I feel that life hasn't forgiven me for treating such treasures with such reckless abandon.

I should've never let her go, because in her—I know now—was that once in a lifetime, lasting love. She was the last girl to see that daring look in my eyes in a way no one would ever see again. Linda saw me the way that I had always wanted to be seen. In her memory is captured a time in my life where I was at the threshold of a most profound change. She took with her—through her life, the David that was surrendered to the hands of fate, the David I will never be again.

And my best friend Dean; I should have stayed with him through it all, until he remembered me once again, as we were before—buddies.

* * *

Instead…the doctor glanced toward my mother with a pensive eye, as his scalpel freed a swollen lymph node from the side of my neck. While holding a part of me in his hand, he pondered for what I felt was a bit too long as we both sat there on the edge of our lives; never more interested in someone else's thoughts than at that very moment. His struggling facial expressions told me all that I needed to know, before his thoughts were able to form words.

Mom appeared to be more optimistic, obviously because I was her son, but I think also not to concern me. Still, I could see her want for relief as she hung on every word, listening for the slightest morsel of hope she might be able to squeeze from this admired professional's opinion.

This decorated doctor was a colleague of hers and a friend as well. My mother was a registered nurse; this made her respect the practice of the medical establishment more often than not without question; only this time she would be denied a prompt answer.

So we left his office where the procedure had taken place, with no "on the record" diagnosis. The lymph node first had to be analyzed, but we all knew that there was a problem. Perhaps more telling were his gestures and the uncomfortable silence between. A conversation of subtle undertones had truly prevailed in the doctor's small office, when we could almost hear each other's heartbeat.

We waited for what seemed like forever. Finally the call came. I was stricken with Hodgkin's disease—cancer of the lymphatic system. It was spreading quickly. By Monday morning a cluster of lymph nodes protruded between my collar bone and the next day on the other side of my neck. It was very scary.

Not much can prepare you for hearing the word cancer when it is directed at you. It's not something I can easily convey, but I will say that it does change a lot of things right away. Your priorities instantly distill themselves to a handful of concerns. There is a sense of urgency in the air that everyone around you feels, but no one feels it more than yourself. True, it was overwhelming news for those who loved me, especially my mother, but it was my life at stake and no other.

From the start, I saw cancer as a one-person trial. It singles out, wielding its dagger under one chin and one chin alone. I never really had any illusions about this. Defending life, for me, was a confronting movement that must begin within me on every level imaginable. I sensed this from the moment I first felt that cold, sharp, instrument, incise my neck, to gather a sample for biopsy.

Cancer can take a mother from her children, a child from a parent, a husband from a wife, a brother or sister from other siblings, or a close friend right from underneath you. In this particular way does it prove to be a one-person trial, though there should never be an underestimation of the power of support. Nonetheless, others can only do so much before they realize life's boundary. They can walk so far with you until life intervenes, letting only one into the arena of trial and tribulation.

When I think back, now that I'm mature enough to appreciate emotional strength in comparison to physical strength, I realize how my mother, who was then on her own with three boys, remained remarkably sturdy through it all. She held it together so well. She stayed just far enough from me to allow me to build my own confidence, yet close enough to let me know that she was there for me. Her ability to balance this was admirably insightful and very much appreciated.

I don't remember a time when I saw worry come across her face. I think this attitude set the tone for our family to deal with what lay ahead for us all. There is no doubt that we were all affected by this. It may have been my battle, but the ramifications were systemic— reaching deep into the core of our family. We were tight and emotionally reliant on each other, so no one really escaped the hurt.

As for me, the delicate balance my mother maintained between strength and allowance had a much more significant impact on my journey. It gave me the freedom to discover what I felt should be discovered on my own. I think my mother understood this, if not outright then intuitively.

I ventured off in another direction, independently, where I could almost see her carefully watch from a distance. I wanted her with me, there was no doubt, but more in the shadow of my lead. I needed to be in possession of my will at that time.

I'm so glad I didn't have to tell her this because I probably wouldn't have. I respected her and I was at times hesitant to go it alone. She could very well have been torn between caring so much for me, and yet sensing my need for this independence, I'll never know for sure. It was clear that I was sailing uncharted waters, having to navigate them with gut feelings. At that point a natural inclination of mine to lead began to take over.

Whether I could see it then or not, this was a time for change. I would need to be much more than what I had been before, because the way I had been before might have actually led me here. I had an even deeper conviction that I would live out once and for all a struggle that had plagued me. It would either take or release me; I was ready for a conclusion, but in no way was I willing to give in.

I wanted the clarity of battle, where there is the action of planning, defending and attacking, followed by a definitive outcome, whatever that might've been. I know that this was a dangerous game, but then again, there was this side of me that needed to make sense of my fears—and life as well.

Maybe I unknowingly allowed this danger, in order to know these truths of life that for some reason seem to elude many of us.

In the days that followed, the underlying fear that I had lived with for so long was not there to greet me in the morning, or tuck me in at night. For some reason, it had left me—entirely. This is how I entered into life's rude den—focused and fearless. Strangely enough, in the face of this unfamiliar territory, I maintained a remarkable steadiness, and possessed a clarity I had not known before. It's true that I stumbled through the beginning as if I was blindfolded.

This is no paradox. The danger was in front of me; the terms were life or death. This could not have been more clear to anyone involved—especially me. At the same time, every move forward was a first. I was in a realm of consequences, and each decision made, whether personal or collective, had the uncertain lingering ahead. I alone would reap the greatest repercussion.

I was a young man caught before so many thresholds, so many realizations, and still I insisted on knowing everything—down to the last detail. I'm not quite sure if this helped or hindered, but I do know that I wouldn't have had it any other way.

I never felt comfortable resting on hope alone; even then it seemed to me a futile gesture. I felt more empowerment being actively involved. Having this kind of attitude, I felt there was a momentum forward, and for me, forward was always a good thing.

I thought about consequences for actions, both inward and outward. I thought about lessons and laws that surpassed what I had learned in life as of yet. These insights came to me briefly, and I didn't spend much time looking into them with any respectable commitment. At that particular time you might say that I was too busy treading water just to stay afloat. But I did have enough sense to take notes when there was a revelation—that is, something discovered that might help me further on. The interesting thing about this was that it wasn't like me to leave a paper trail. It was the first time writing meant anything to me. I felt as if what I was going through was worth noting. So, instinctively I jotted everything down that helped me get by. What was happening to me was powerful enough to completely change my life. If I didn't grab hold of the reins of this runaway predicament I was in, I knew that I would be in serious trouble.

In the beginning, I placed my fate directly in the hands of the doctors. In my eyes they were gods; although something made me feel uneasy about such an absolute compliance, for no reason other than it wasn't my nature. I followed their lead like a good little boy who takes his medicine without spilling a drop. I really had no choice. After all, I was a guest in their world of expertise, and the hospital was their domain.

I hadn't yet experienced the downsides of these relied-upon therapies, nor did I completely understand the tradeoffs I was in for just to buy me precious time. In their world, combating cancer conventionally is a slow evolution, both in thought and application. Modern medicine treats the whole of a society in the best way that it knows how—with a broad stroke, but I believe the truth of health eludes the medical establishment's grasp exactly because of this.

In this particular theater, where the manifestation of cancer is as unique as the person it invades, the only true course medicine must take is an individual one, with a whole body approach where a complete dissection of relating entities within the individual is scrutinized for imbalances. Doctors would need to see the patient with a much more encompassing perspective, and the patient would need to be more involved with this new method.

At sixteen years old, those thoughts hadn't yet occurred to me, so I followed the standard as only I knew how, which ultimately left me fully bound to this engagement—destined to stumble awkwardly through these moments of uncertainty.

So at the age of sixteen I prepared for a protocol tailored to treat Hodgkin's disease. The first assault on my body began within days of my initial biopsy. An exploratory laparotomy operation was performed in order to stage the progression of the cancer. In the process, my spleen was removed because it too had disease. I was fortunate that it hadn't reached my liver, which brought the staging to 3a instead of 3b. The staging is done from one to four, with the letters A and B as sublevels within these numbers. 3A was a later stage of the disease, but anymore than this would've been very serious; it would've meant the liver was affected as well. Stage four would mean that the bone marrow was involved; a grave prognosis.

There were signs of cancer throughout my torso, from my neck to my groin. It had spread very quickly in a short amount of time. After a meeting between the doctors, my parents, and me, we reached an agreement to first treat with radiation. I knew nothing about this therapy, but took their advice that it was the best choice. The other alternative was chemotherapy, to which, we were told, Hodgkin's disease was less responsive.

There seemed to be an urgency to get on with treatments. Our decision was made with the best knowledge we had at the time, forgoing a second opinion. From the description of these therapies, as they were explained to us, picking one over the other was a choice of lesser evils; both were caustic.

With my suture still healing, the doctors went ahead, delivering the first dose of radiation two weeks later. There was no turning back now. Years ago, radiation was given more generally than it is today, that is, in a less precise method. In this limited respect we have come a long way, but fine tuning these types of therapies doesn't get around the fact that we are not where we should be in medicine. To me, poison is poison, whether in small doses or large; it still destroys healthy cells as well. But we have to use what is at our disposal, regardless of the side effects.

Its effects on me were evident, as I started vomiting within hours of returning home from the clinic; I vomited until there was nothing but dry heaves. Not until the late evening or early morning after did I want to eat anything, and even at that point I was still unusually particular about what I wanted.

Not long after, my hair began falling out, leaving large amounts on my pillow in the morning and in my hands as I washed it. In time, I began dreading Tuesdays' because that was the day of the week I would have to go to the radiology department and sit with people often ten times my age. I stood out there like a refreshing anomaly. Some would just stare. I wasn't sure why, nor was I the least bit bothered; I thought it might have something to do with my youth, so I always smiled back politely.

I often thought about them too, wondering if they were a bit apprehensive, or frightened even. I knew we were all there basically for the same reason. While each of us endured our own struggles on a very personal level, there was this common thread imperceptibly connecting our plights. I think we were comforted by each other's company.

I felt weaker and weaker as the treatments piled up, losing so much weight that I had to stop weighing myself because I was becoming increasingly disheartened. No longer did I recognize the football player or the wrestler that I once was. The only thing that mattered now was not feeling nauseated. I withdrew from seeing my friends for fear they would not recognize me. I couldn't bear this realization. Strangers were fine, because they never knew me before this. But the thought of seeing such surprised looks on the faces of friends who had admired my strength concerned me. I was an immeasurable distance from my friends and it made no sense for me to drag them there too. I never explained this to anyone; I just hoped they would understand.

As the days of recovery passed, and the treatments were in process, my life began to transform physically and emotionally—but not yet spiritually. The only way that I really knew this person I was becoming was by the reflection of my relation with my mother. She was nearest to me through it all, and so I looked to her for acknowledgement in many ways. After all, who better to guide me than one who loves me the most? Who better to trust in, than the one who would sacrifice her own life for mine? Who better to relate with the world than the one who delivered me here? Clearly, mom would be my confidant and no other would do, because she had this strength. I cannot imagine having gone through this without her, and I'm so glad I didn't have to.

The effects from the harsh therapy began to take its toll. I started experiencing repeated attacks of enteritis from the radical radiation I received to my intestinal area. My first episode came three months into the course. It was severe enough to bring me into the emergency room.

After being admitted, I was diagnosed with acute radiation enteritis, and given the appropriate medicine for pain, while an IV dripped fluids to keep me hydrated. It was a good two weeks before I felt well enough to go home, but I was faced with the possibility of this coming back, which gave me apprehension.

No one was familiar with radiation enteritis at that time. The specialists were very interested in these findings because the occurrence was rare, especially when treating Hodgkin's disease. This warranted further investigation. I would be monitored closely during the remaining doses given.

The oncologist was intent on completing my last course of treatment as soon as possible. I had one more four-week run ahead of me, so I braced myself one more time and followed protocol. Therapy ended shortly after my birthday in April. I looked ahead with a sense of jubilation. The summer was on its way and the long winter had finally passed. I spent the first few months trying very hard to put some weight back on. It was a grueling effort. I was very tired with just a limited amount of energy to disperse.

Preparing and making each meal proved taxing, but I was determined to eat only nutritious foods, because I saw the importance of this right from the beginning. Mom was working sixteen-hour days to keep a roof over our head. Louis was in college and living at our father's house, which wasn't too far away. Tommy was in school during the day. This left me on my own to cope.

I couldn't bring myself to socialize with anyone outside of my family; I didn't have that confidence—in myself or in my condition. I drifted from those bonds that had meant so much to me, just short of a year ago. I don't think I really understood what I was doing or how much I would miss everyone who initially tried to stay in touch with me.

Time was unforgiving; I never retrieved this loss.

My only distraction from the distance I created between the life I had known and the life emerging was attempting to restore my physical health to something close to what I once knew. This kept me from complete discouragement. My body had been ravaged. I wasn't tending to a sprained ankle or a sore throat, it was much more than this; I could not treat it as such. To heal in this manner required a level of depth, discipline and patience that I was not ready for. Those were frustrating times to be sure, but I was determined to see my way through.

I took an interest in medical literature. Fortunately, my mother had kept most of her books from college, and my father saved his as well. Hers was knowledge about the physical body, and the books he possessed, having had a master's in psychology, was knowledge in human behavior. Both aspects held my attention. They were insightful. I learned all that I could, but there was something missing from this type of knowledge. I felt as if I was learning about the stars and the planets but not what force held them there. That's really what I wanted to know about; what it was behind the mystery of whatever brings the harmony of health to a body. That would intrigue me! I was compelled to find the answer.

My need to know kept leading me in another direction. There was mystery swirling wonderfully, powerfully, around me, and a quiet urgency that wouldn't leave me alone—not then, not ever. In time it lead me away from all that we know—all that I knew. These were pieces to a greater puzzle in life beyond our traditions, our customs, and petty knowledge—not readily found in literature; important pieces that cannot easily be captured and then bound where dust can settle between the pages. There is a living intelligence which exists beyond this, and I was being made aware of its presence. The more I leaned in this direction the more it drew me closer.

These were only brief moments of clarity that would send a rush right through me, as if I had momentarily realized God. It's so hard to hang on to such a promise when it is so unfamiliar, and also when you are going through an experience which almost continuously tests your resolve. But it is exactly these times that bring exceptional opportunity to the surface of your consciousness, when there is not a moment to spare for shallow thoughts to occupy your mind. I know that I had no room for shallow thoughts. I wanted to think about these things.

The end of summer was upon me and I had gained back a considerable amount of weight by diligence and desire, a combination that, for me, would reap results. I felt comfortable with myself once again, and I had managed to layer a feeling of achievement somewhere between the many layers of emotions I experienced towards my ordeal, albeit a very thin layer. I made the most of this confidence when it came to me. It was right about that time that I received an invitation to hang out with an old friend of mine. I hadn't heard from him for many months. We were childhood friends later separated by schools and it was only the summer breaks that would bring us together. He had heard that I was on my way to recovering and contacted me to see if I was up to a day out with some other friends I hadn't seen in a while. I felt great anticipation after ending my treatments in the early spring. After a bit of hesitancy I accepted. When he picked me up I asked where we were headed. He spoke of a get-together near the beach; a final fling with freedom before school's opening bell.

I put aside my vanity and apprehension because I wanted a change of scenery, and because I really felt like seeing people. I think that I may have talked myself into believing I could go on as if nothing had happened. I had a moment of "what the heck," swirling around in my bag of possibles, and I reached for it. The idea of normality was enticing, and in the end, won over my reluctance.

It was great seeing everyone there and I forgot for the moment everything that I had been through. Someone offered me a beer and I saw nothing wrong with this indulgence; after all, I deserved the pleasure and was having a good time.

A short time later I started to feel a slight pain in my gut. It was familiar to the one I had when the enteritis first came to me. I dismissed it, hoping it would subside but it didn't; instead it intensified. I knew then that I was in trouble and I was a long way from home and, more importantly, the hospital. I had made a mistake. How much I would pay for it was still up in the air. By now, my friend could see that there was a problem. I did all that I could to downplay the symptoms, but he knew we needed to do something quickly. There comes a point when you don't care anymore about hiding the pain, because it's much too distracting to front; I was past that point. My friend realized that he had to get me home as fast as possible.

What I had feared was happening; I was bringing a good friend into my personal war and there was nothing I could do about it now; it was done. We slipped out of the party without notice, hopped in his car and raced for home. We were still a good distance from my house and I was doubled over in pain. I can't imagine what was going through his mind at the time. This was exactly why I had chosen not to venture out or invite anyone in, because my condition was too unpredictable and outside of my control.

I remember on the way back, we had stopped for a red light; I couldn't sit still and literally got out of the car, falling to my knees and then crashing to the pavement. He kept telling me it would be all right and that we'd be home soon; I barely heard him but managed to crawl back in. By the time we reached the driveway of my house the car door was already open and I fell out to the curb. I passed out and came to as I dashed for the front door. My mother had seen me through the living room window and met me in the doorway. I tried my best to explain what was happening to me but the pain prevented this and again I collapsed the floor.

I was helpless.

Tommy jumped out and held me up while we rushed to the car. They literally had to drag me in. When I think about how my younger brother needed to hold up his bigger brother, I can't say what that felt like to me; I would much rather forget it.

We finally arrived at the emergency room, where we rushed in like gangbusters. I was admitted right away and eventually brought to a room divided by curtains. Realizing that I wasn't alone, but in a four-person room, fully occupied, I moaned under my breath so no one could hear me.

One day became two, two became three—then I stopped keeping track. By the first week, my abdomen extended out as if I was nine months pregnant. A tube was placed in my nose to drain the bile and poisons from my stomach. Because of the empty calories in IV sugar water, my weight plummeted; I moved even further towards emaciation.

After a week of extreme agony, I wasn't "deflating," only getting worse. I often looked down at my stomach and wondered what was happening inside me.

Emotionally, I was just getting by. There's nothing like seeing the best doctors not know what to do. It kind of teaches you to not rely so much on them but find a sense of calm within. I began to realize that I would have a much greater threshold of defiance over death than they could ever give me. After all, it was my life in the balance.

The doctors believed I had a slim chance of survival, and expressed this to my mother. The only option would be to operate immediately before my intestines burst inside me, which would have poisoned me. My mother could not make this decision, so I made it for her. They gave me a fifty-fifty chance of surviving the operation, but the odds were less had I stayed on my present course of lay and wait.

The doctors just weren't sure what the outcome would be; there wasn't any 'been there done that' experience to draw from. There were very few cases then of radiation enteritis to reference.

I was hurried into surgery. I don't remember a thing about that day, not even waking up.

After the operation the surgeon informed my mother that three feet of the small intestine had been severely burned, twisted and obstructed and that it was dangerously close to rupturing. Fortunately, he didn't remove any of my guts. He claimed that it was salvageable, and also a crucial portion of the bowels, where much of the nutrients we get from food were absorbed.

That decision—though I am very grateful that he made it—has brought me into the emergency room numerous times through the years, experiencing bouts of intolerable pain, only to be relieved by medication, rest and a liquid diet. Having this condition has taught me to have patience with myself. I've learned how to cope with gaining—then losing, then gaining back and so on. I was beginning to adjust to this unpredictable future. It wasn't easy, in fact it was downright frustrating, but I wasn't one to complain about things I couldn't change. I just tried even harder to overcome. I'm a believer in conviction.

School had begun classes and I was not there to attend my senior year, but instead was tutored at home by a wonderful girl named Amy. It took months to fully recover from the surgery, but even longer to gain back all the weight I had lost in the process. Losing so much weight made me very weak. It was a slow progression back to feeling better in any way, but I was improving. I refused to let this get the best of me or discourage me in any way.

The new winter had snuck up on me, keeping me inside for many months. I was always cold because I was so thin. I didn't like being cooped up for so long without getting some fresh air. I would rather have gone to my grandfather's farm and lost myself in the dense woods where no thought of being sick could ever follow me. My brothers and I spent many weekends there as kids, with my cousins, running waywardly through the well trodden trails, and even further inward to a fresh-flowing brook that naturally divided the properties. There were deep, clear, golden pools offset from the running water, with glimmering sand that almost looked like speckles of glistening gold layering the bottom. This—from reflections of the sun that maneuvered around the grand, skyscraping, pines—canopying the very old, manmade, stonewalls, which sliced through and crisscrossed our crude playground. We called this area of the woods the dark forest, because the massive pines would partially eclipse the sun, even in midday. It was there that we hadn't a care in the world. We could be a few hundred yards deep and feel like we were stranded in the wilderness somewhere in the Adirondacks, or the foothills of the Smoky Mountains. Our imagination had no boundaries. It was our retreat from the structured world that was beginning to mold us.

More than ever—I needed this now, but I would have to be patient. I wasn't ready to venture. I could say then that I knew exactly what cabin fever felt like. I held more reservations than ever of leaving my home to see anyone or be anywhere else for any length of time.

It was late spring and the warmth had finally thawed New England. I found enough confidence to attend the final days of school with my class, and was blessed enough to actually graduate with them. I would even be present at the ceremony as well. Initially, there was an air of awkwardness in the classrooms whenever anyone saw me. The mood was unusually quiet, I think because no one really knew how to act or what to say. We were all too young to maneuver around the obvious—present company included.

I didn't feel nearly the same anymore; I felt like I stuck out. There was something about me that had changed, I believe, much more than physically, and I was hoping no one had noticed. I wanted to be so far away from there and never look back again. I think life separated me from my peers in such a way that I had no idea how to get back to them. It had changed me from within as well as without. I didn't understand this then as much as I do now.

A very small part of me did fit in though, and it was just enough to appreciate youth's closing window of opportunity. I had to join my classmates one last time before we were dispersed to our fateful places in a society waiting patiently for us to fill them.

Following graduation, my spirits were high and my outlook towards the future remained tentatively optimistic. But life seldom considers feelings, desires or plans. Most often it has its own course it sets you on.

I was barely eighteen in the early summer of '82. The ink on my high school diploma hadn't yet dried and I was again admitted to Rhode Island Hospital—what had turned out to be my home away from home—this time to weather shingles. My hope of a sustaining remission from cancer had been crushed. I had just begun a course of chemotherapy, a little more than a year and a half after enduring radical radiation treatments for Hodgkin's disease that caused me some major problems. Sometimes I wonder why I even agreed to it to begin with. A thought of regret creeps into my consciousness before I am able to admonish it. I cannot change the past. I must remember this.

A relapse swings me full circle. I can't believe that I'm right back where I started.

In the shower I noticed a swelling under my left arm pit. It just didn't feel right to me. I had those same feelings when I first found a swollen lymph node on the side of my neck. But then I was young and fresh for the battle, eager to take on this fight. All that has happened to me has managed to smother what little fire still burns within. Nonetheless, I have no choice in my mind but to do what must be done. I'm still willing to press on undaunted, because I know what awaits me should I give up. I know the silent decision lingering ever present, that must never be made until all active hope is exhausted. No one speaks openly of this decision, but that doesn't mean it's not tucked away in the back of each our minds, ready to be rendered on any given day, at any given moment. It's our last bit of freedom over our lives that we protect, to show death that we have the final say. Even in the presence of finality—we rebel. I was never able to admit this to myself. One day I would have to come to terms with dying. So much energy was spent fearing this aspect of life. I didn't understand what place death had in my life, and this made living tentative and awkward.

The new treatment of chemotherapy caused my white blood count to drop below 500, leaving me vulnerable to a host of life threatening infections. It was during this time that Tommy had come home from summer school one day, unaware of the passenger he'd brought along. Of course it wasn't his fault. How could he know of this intruder that was much too small to see? He carried with him a fairly common virus capable of leaving only superficial scars in healthy kids, but second and third degree layers of skin torn and fleshy in someone with a compromised immune system—someone like me.

Tommy mentioned to our mother that some of the kids at school had chickenpox. I could see her face as she made the connection and realized the danger. But we both know now there was nothing we could've done then. Within forty-eight hours of this news, I began showing signs of infection. Fortunately, mom had the sense to rush me to the emergency room as soon as we noticed patches of circular burns developing across my waist. I began feeling intense pain in my side, just to the right of my navel. It soon traveled around to my spine, and by then the clusters of burns began to connect, forming one massive, fleshy wound, fully encompassing my whole right side, from my navel to my spine.

I was on a stretcher placed in a crowded corridor. The emergency room stalls were fully occupied. My mother held my hand as I gently squeezed hers from the pain. She never let go. She was there with me the whole time. Her eyes calmed me. It would be the last time for two agonizing days I saw her or anyone else that I loved.

It wasn't long before the doctors told my mother that I had contracted a bad case of shingles. What made matters even worse was that it began disseminating unchallenged, throughout my whole body. Things started to become surreal as movement around me quickened.

Before I knew what hit me, I was taken on a stretcher quietly through the empty halls in the late night hour, where I was wheeled past two nurses already waiting for me in this private corner room on the third floor of Jane Brown Hospital. It was a special section of Rhode Island Hospital, reserved for surgery, cancer and isolated patients, along with other provisional circumstances that I'm not fully aware of. The orderly laid me on top of a crisp, somewhat sterile linen sheet and left noticeably hastily, realizing that he was the only one in the room not wearing a mask.

I wasn't at all familiar with shingles, nor did I know what to expect. I was aware that there were very concerned eyes staring back at me. No one settled me or told me then that I will be all right; whether I needed that comfort or not, it was not offered.

It was early morning, the night had passed, but I hadn't slept a wink. I was wide-eyed and trembling, not from fear, but from excruciating pain searing through my nerve endings, and penetrating the surrounding tissue.

I was left alone for many hours without doctors or nurses, while set back the furthest from any other room on the wing. There were moments I thought that I might've been forgotten. It was so quiet where I was that I could barely hear the sound of life beyond the threshold of my doorway. It was during such times that the mind can wear us down if we let it, but can also take on a new strength if we insist on it.

I was a world away from the casual liberties of someone my own age. The walls around me were stripped bare of the immaterial, a stark reflection of the patient within them. There was no place there for vanity. It was one of the first things my mind let go of. There were much more important issues to be concerned with. Something that I couldn't see or understand was trying its best to overcome me. I was living each moment, knowing that I was in the fight of my life; a hope of many more sunsets to see, or eternal darkness was at stake before me.

If I was fortunate, I stole—from my aggressor—fifteen minutes or so of shut-eye. I was later punished for this morsel as I woke to a living nightmare, straining with every bit of strength I had inside of me to ward off the pain. The first two nights I spent alone, without any of my family. The days seemed to have almost passed with a sense of strange vagueness. I didn't remember them at all. All that I saw were eyes behind masks and gowns, entering now and then, to look after my newly emerging wounds.

The shingles was spreading all over my body, and beginning to cover my face. Between intense itching and the deep, nagging pain, it was pure torture. The medical staff had no idea that the medication they dutifully gave me brought little relief, and I was too distracted to think of this; it just didn't occur to me. I knew that the meds were given every two hours, so it must have helped me in some way. I can say now that I was severely under-medicated; I have no doubt of this. No one knew enough then to do a proper pain assessment. I'm certain that I never had a full evaluation in that room, and suffered greatly because of this, much more than I should have.

I would see my mother first, and then my father, as he followed her in the room. They were no longer together, but a dying son made them overlook any irreconcilable differences they might've had.

I never saw them really—just their eyes, but that was enough to satisfy me. I drifted in and out of consciousness from both the excruciating pain and the fact that I hadn't had a decent rest in days. I remember catching myself coming in and out of this realm of consciousness. I distinctly can see my father sitting across the bed, watching me, as my eyes reflected this inner journey. The brief moments of my lucidity presented an opportunity for him to inquire if I was alright. I nodded in affirmation. Then he would tell me to stop scratching my face or I would scar. I was doing all that I could not to rip my skin off with my fingernails.

I knew that he thought the worst. I could see that concerned look on his face. He didn't recognize this person lying in bed right in front of him. He couldn't hide this from me. It was not the David that he had watched swiftly conquer his opponents with a natural ability.

If he only knew that I was in the midst of realizing my own salvation, that at times I was so far away from my stricken flesh and without any thought of being afraid of what was to come of me. If only he could see that I was still there within my nearly beaten and battered body.

That same spirit that imposed its will upon competitors had not retreated. I think if he had searched my eyes, he would have known this; this might've given him hope.

At one point when he thought that I wasn't paying attention, I saw him motion to my mother to look at my neck when it tensed up from the pain, where they could see every pronounced vein. My mother wiped the sweat that dripped from my forehead with a face cloth saturated with cool water as tears welled in her eyes. I was trying so hard not to show her how much pain I was in, but there was no way to conceal it.

In her eyes I could see what love would look like if it was a tangible thing. I wanted to tell her so much that I loved her too but I knew that she already knew this.

It was time to go home, as visiting hours ended. This left me a bit relieved, even though I would miss them; because alone, I was able to retreat to an inner place that I discovered, where I was taken far away from the moment. It was there that I let my mind wander free. It is there that I was delivered from the immobility of lying in bed. Earlier thoughts and dreams were dying right before me and new ones were

fast emerging. I had an empty canvas to paint a picture of my immediate desires; one of which was to feast on juicy watermelon and sweet,
strawberries. Simple pleasures, yet so far from my lips.

In my mind, against the sky, a movie screen played back the most
memorable times of my life, and this would sustain me. I stayed far
away from the present for as long as I was able; in no way from fear or
denial, but because there was nothing passionate or inspiring around
me. In my retreat there were times when I would see my closest
friends in the distance, though I did not run to them, because I knew
better; I knew that I was there in thought only. Then a voice inter-
vened. It told me that I might not ever reach them again. I stood and
watched with neither sadness nor envy, until they all faded away, and I
was once again back in my room.

I thought of the future in terms of hours, and even minutes, which
seemed to work for me; it was the way it should be. I told myself that if
I could make it through the minutes, then the hours will naturally
follow. I need not be concerned with the days or beyond that. Such
apprehension would've been wasted energy, and could only lead to fear.

*It had been many days since I first laid my head on that pillow; no, more like
weeks*—I wondered. My only means to glimpse life beyond that room
was through the window across from me. Outside of that great
window, I saw hints of summer in the courtyard, where one, two, or
maybe three trees managed to thrive between buildings. It was a
beautiful sight for my sore eyes, to see such new and tender leaves
against the contrasting structures of brick and mortar. It brought to
me a feeling of fresh anticipation and evoked a faint desperation,
which overcame me at times. I knew that the seasons would again
escape me without my notice, without me having really lived them. I
knew they would leave no lasting impressions of a crisp beginning or
definitive end. I knew this because I had lived it before. I was familiar
with the disparity of time as it passed in my room and outside where
the world went on. *Would I ever live the seasons again?* I wondered.

It seemed that in that room time had slowed as still as a sail hung its lowest in a dead calm. But outside, nothing waited for me; it went on with or without me. It was there that I learned how temporal our presence can be.

The nurses ran their shifts as they passed the baton to one another, with eager thoughts of returning home to their loved ones, and life far from we who were not well. Even the janitor was free to leave at some point, though I wasn't envious, only appreciative of the brief company.

While I was there, I began to sense a connection to greater things much more than myself. In fact, there were many new sensations that both plagued me and brought me confidence. I wasn't sure what was going on or what this signified, but there was definitely a sense that was new to me, making its presence known. Even though my life was so close to death, I had never felt so alive; I had never been so aware of life. I was in a zone. My spirit was overriding my mind and keeping it steady and on course. I was just eighteen years old and isolated from all that I knew, with no real defense that one could point to for certainty, yet I was finding that I wasn't alone at all.

In fact, I was in the presence of intelligence, with the company of humanity by my side. All that was required of me was to believe in life, in myself; to focus on the moment and not to let my emotions overtake me. The rest would come to me.

I could do this. I wanted to live. I wouldn't let anything take life away from me without a fight. I believed that no matter what happened in that room, I had the final say; not only did I believe this, but I knew it.

The shingles had reached the lids of my eyes, and they were telling my parents that I would soon be blind. Nowhere on my body was the skin clear of this virus.

At one point, a team of doctors who I had never seen before came into the room to ask my permission to take pictures of my condition.

They wanted to use this occurrence in text as an extreme case of shingles outbreak. I consented.

I'm certain somewhere out there sits on a shelf the evidence of what I lived through; though I'm not sure I would ever want to see this.

If ever there was a scent of death in the air, it would have to have been in my hospital room. Somewhere in the midst of that stench, I was barely surviving—pressed hard against life and death, each tugging at me with a very deliberate intention. I could feel every bit of their touch, of their need for an outcome—either way. Their breath breathed right through me when my body rested and held when it strained. Life and death was pulling my emotions both ways and savagely tearing at my will, reminding me that no one could save me from their purpose. I must fight to stay alive, I self-affirmed.

In the end, I knew that it would be my choice, whether or not I would give in. This determination kept me on a razor's edge of awareness, while I tried my hardest to make heads or tails of it all. I kept reminding myself that I had only to see my way through the minutes. That's all I needed to do. Looking at it this way was doable.

All the while, beads of sweat continued to trickle from my forehead, as I strained to bear the pain that ripped through my side. Every chance to remember whatever good thoughts I could retrieve, I took. I tried to inspire myself the best way that I knew how, before the pain yanked me back to reality. *I have made it so far.* I thought. *Anything is possible. Nothing could take my life while I was watching; I wouldn't let it.* I confronted this hostility against me and defied it. Every minute I survived bolstered my tenacity. *How dare you try to steal my life when I haven't even lived yet! What right do you have?*

If this was not a time to be dramatic, then when would've been? Nothing stirred my willpower more than injustice. That was a time to reinforce my will or I might have run the risk of letting my guard down and succumbing. I needed to be sending messages to myself, reinforcing my dominance over this threat. Considering what I was up against, I believe nothing short of this would have worked.

Visiting hours had passed once again, and I noticed that my father had left on schedule. My mother remained by my side, unable to separate herself from me, because she knew something that I didn't. That may have been true, but I was living through something that she could never understand, which was much more relevant. The doctor told her that it might be days if not hours, but the end was inevitable. There was nothing more they could do. It appeared the shingles virus had a firm grip on my body and it wouldn't let go. It was doing what it was meant to do. That was how it survived.

I kept telling myself that if I could make it through the night and then through the next day, then I would get through this eventually. I was doing what I had to do—to survive.

Mom was convinced by the staff to go home for the night. I lay quiet while she left; my eyes followed hers out the door. She paused near the doorway, looked back to me one last time, and then she was gone.

It was after midnight, the air was stifling. The nurse came in to medicate me. She noticed that I was not coherent, and proceeded to feel my forehead. She left the room in a hurry, and soon returned with a thermometer in hand. She waited as I scorched the mercury-filled glass. *What was happening to me? I didn't feel right at all.* Another nurse followed in to take my blood, and then she was gone. It wasn't long before the house doctor arrived with his team. It was very late for this visit and unusual. His words were matter-of-fact and direct. He spoke to me while everyone watched me from behind him.

"David, can you understand me?" I nodded to him in affirmation, but said nothing. "You have a bacterial infection in your blood. Your temperature is 105 degrees. We need your permission to treat you with antibiotics right away. There is no time for delay."

Between all the medication in my system, the dangerously high temperature I had, my extreme pain, and the unusual dire nature of his delivery, I grew paranoid; I actually thought that they had come into my room for one purpose—to put me out of my misery. My first impulse was to sidestep and negotiate around his intentions. I felt trapped by his 'do or die' scenario. I stalled them with redundant questions, but he had an answer for everything, which frustrated me. He told me that there was no time to contact my doctor or my parents; he told me that I needed to give him the OK.

What I really needed in this state of mind was some time to work this out; I was delusional. I asked them to leave the room momentarily; they reluctantly agreed. He told me that they would be right outside, but he would need an answer soon. I acknowledged. I asked him to close the door on the way out. They were gone.

I have a moment of freedom! I thought, in relief. I then looked around the room for ways to escape. My first thought was to tie the bed sheets together and shimmy out of the window, down three floors. The window was fixed, thick, and tempered glass, so this idea was quickly abandoned. The only other way out was through the door they had just left. This was much more reasonable—even for a desperado. I climbed out of my bed for the first time since I was brought into the room, wearing a jonnie and nothing else, weighing no more than a hundred and five pounds soaking wet. I was burning up with fever and I had raw flesh, bandaged, from my navel to my spine. The rest of me was covered with disseminating shingles—and I wanted to escape!

I snuck quietly to the door and cracked it open enough to see what was outside; the coast was clear. I ventured out a little further to see the nurses' station, where the medical team waited patiently. It was a good twenty or so yards away. *This was my chance.* I figured. There was an elevator just across the hall. I dashed for the down button like some less than noble caped crusader. I heard someone call out, "He's leaving!" The door opened and I jumped in.

I made it, now what? I thought. My heart was pounding right through my chest. *Ok, when I get downstairs I'll hail a taxi and it will take me home.* I tried to plan. Then suddenly the elevator doors reopened on the second floor; I was startled to see three or four people rush in to grab me. I resisted them—then passed out.

I awakened to see many around my bedside, reminiscent of Dorothy in "The Wizard of Oz"; only they were not here to comfort me. I was told that I had lost valuable time, and that my parents were on their way. I finally gave in to their requests. Antibiotics were administered soon after.

It was nearly two in the morning and my mother and father arrived. They looked very worried for me; though my father's eyes exposed a much grimmer outlook for me. I understood; it was who he was. He saw things as they were. There was no mystery to hold to for him, only what the doctors told him would be, just what was there in front of him to see. I didn't say anything about what had just happened, but I was sure they already knew.

As things settled down, and they saw that I was out of immediate danger, my father suggested they both go home to get some rest. He told my mother that she could come back in the morning. They requested a private nurse to stay by my side, to watch me, so I didn't try again to escape.

She wasted no time and changed my dressings as a precautionary measure, to prevent further infection. The energy exerted in my attempt to escape left me exhausted, and I finally fell asleep.

I knew my mother was making peace with this. She was one to reach for prayer in trying times. What better time would there ever be than right then—when she was so close to losing her middle son? I'm quite sure she told God that my life was in his hands. She was emotionally overwhelmed and lent my fate to the heavens. She knew that God would do whatever was best for me. She was all right with that. She didn't want me to suffer any longer. If that heavy emotional burden was lifted from her shoulders, then I was all right with that. My mother had been much more than my rock; she had been to me every bit of what a mother should ever be. In my eyes she was the nearest thing to God.

Long gone were the simple cares of the day that I once had; simplicity that may partly be ode to the leniencies of life, if there was such a thing. How well it casts its mirth upon the sun-dried smile of a still-seasoning youth—when all things are right! What was it that you whispered to me ever so gently, when I wasn't listening—when I thought I had forever ahead of me? I wonder now, will I have another chance to live? Will life allow me a second wind? Will it show me a way through this?

UP FROM THE ASHES

Where one does—many can, and all is possible.

I t was peaceful that morning after. The nurses stayed clear of my room. There were no early morning interruptions. My eyes had not yet opened to the natural light that came gently unnoticed into my room, but inside there remained the radiance of a thousand suns. I still had so much life left in me.

A hand touched my forehead, startling me. I glanced to my side where the nurse sat waiting for me to awaken, her eyes warm and compassionate. She was a reminder of what had happened through the night, that it was real and not some nightmare. I needed so much to see her face right then. The one thing that brought me comfort was to watch her mask wrinkle briefly from a hidden smile. At that moment I was certain that I had made it.

Strangely, I felt energy that I hadn't had in weeks. Something changed within me—of this I am sure. The pain had lessened and I became aware enough to remember what had recently happened to me. I reflected on the last few days at first, and then before that. It was sobering. It was as if I had awakened from another time and place; somewhere I would never want to be again.

For the first time since being there I felt restless. In my thoughts I wandered beyond the confines of my bed, beyond what I had endured. There was clarity of the moment that I cannot explain, but if I had to, I might say that I was fully conscious of my surroundings. They appeared to me as never before. It was as if time had begun to pass once again—in my room.

I had a sense of freedom that was once restrained by pain, medicine and high fever. I was desperate to move about in some way, and would even settle for a few steps just outside of my room. I made up my mind to do just that.

As I lifted myself from the bed, the nurse followed every move until I had gotten to my feet. I looked in her eyes, attempting a smile as she nodded in affirmation, still not having said a word. She trusted that I knew what I was doing, and I was not looking for permission; I was determined. After taking a few steps with her support, I let go as she followed me out the door. I needed this. These were very liberating times for me. It might have been a little early to claim such independence, considering my recent attempt to escape, that now seemed to me—quite embarrassing. But things were different this time; I had my senses.

I paced myself down the hall just far enough to peek inside a few rooms. I remember making eye contact with each patient as I walked by; I wouldn't look away until they acknowledged me. I wanted them to know they were not alone. The only thing separating us were walls surrounding our beds. We all were not well—together. I wanted to show them that I was all right. Maybe they would feel that confidence or see it in my eyes, I wasn't sure, but at least I could try. It felt so natural for me to extend myself in this way. I didn't think about how they would perceive me, or whether they really gave a damn. That wasn't as important as my connecting with them.

This was an attitude so out of character for me. When I played sports, I thought singularly. At times I even had to be reminded that I was on a team. I was devoted to everyone I played with but I never really grasped this "team player" concept. I figured if I did well then my team would in turn benefit. This time, it wasn't whether or not we won a game, the stakes were much higher. My experiences with death so far showed me how serious life can be, and also how precious it is as well.

I was beginning to feel a relation to others on a deeper level. There *was* life beyond myself; I wanted to reach out to it just then. That want might very well have been a hint of what lay ahead for me.

Time spent away from my room was brief but rejuvenating. My steps began to waver as sweat spilled from my brow. I felt lightheaded. I started to favor one side, leaning over to my right side as I walked back. Every step caused me to wince, reminding me why I was there in the first place.

I then heard a voice behind me, a voice that I have heard all of my life, but which never sounded better. It was my mother, frozen there with wonder and disbelief as she watched her son steadily standing on his own. I will always remember her reaction.

"David! You're OK, my God!" I turned around. She hurried toward me in tears. I stood there, barely able to smile, as frail as one can be, waiting until she had reached me. I couldn't take another step. I let her hug me for as long as she needed to. I was too weak to grab hold of her, so in her arms we embraced.

My mother couldn't understand. By all accounts things should have gotten worse, not better. I don't think anyone completely understood what was happening. Instead of dying, I was starting to live again. The tide had shifted in the direction of life. I'm sure that I surprised the nurses as well. They watched me suffer for weeks and most likely prayed that it would end. But did they see this promise of life deep within me? Did they know who I was or what guided me through—hidden way beneath the surface? They were much like my mother, under the influence of a profession that conditioned them to look at illness as a process of predictability. But what they witnessed that day didn't fit this perception. None of this made sense in the medical field. Yet it was happening right in front of their eyes, right in front of my mother—in a controlled environment no less.

My mother's disbelief quickly turned to acceptance as the mother side of her won over logic. It was the first time in a long time I had seen her smile and really mean it. She couldn't help but cry because of the immense joy that overwhelmed her. I have never seen my mother so happy than at that very moment, the instant she realized her son just might live. It was no small victory in this great battle in the course of a dreadful war against cancer.

Mom hadn't slept well for days, if not weeks, and I knew that she needed to catch up if we were going to get through the rest of this together. I was finally able to send her home after promising her that I would be in the same condition if not better when she returned. I believed this.

Later that afternoon, I got an unexpected visit from my doctor. He was a family friend, and the chief hematologist in the Department of Hematology at Rhode Island Hospital. I liked this doctor very much. I felt comfortable in his presence. He was an unassuming, gentle man who chose his words carefully, because I think he realized how literal they could be in a situation such as mine.

I was delighted to see him because I wanted to share my good news, but I sensed that he had already heard. Maybe this is why he came to see me at such an unusual time. His visits were periodic at best because of his hectic schedule, and they usually took place at night. I noticed he was without a mask this time, letting me know that he had been told that I was feeling much better. He made his way around the bed to my left arm where within my armpit could be found cancerous lymph nodes. He went straight for it.

While talking to me, he lifted my arm and began to probe underneath as his questions brought back the reality of my situation. That was the first time since I'd been admitted for shingles that my cancer had been brought up at all. I had almost forgotten about it myself with everything else that was happening. Actually, no one had monitored its progress since I had been in isolation. I don't think it ever occurred to anyone till now.

As the doctor examined me with my arm slightly elevated, he asked if I had received any treatments while I was here. *Shouldn't you know; you are my doctor?* I thought to myself. I answered respectfully that I hadn't been treated since I was in the clinic weeks ago. It was a fact that I was much too weak for this kind of therapy. I think he realized this but was a little perplexed by what he had found, or not found. He now had my attention and suddenly my breathing slowed as the room quieted. I didn't say a word after. I watched him closely and waited.

There it was—I caught a glimpse of a peculiar expression. He seemed almost mystified.

But why would he be mystified? He was a professional. I thought. I knew that he was probing the site for signs of cancer, but why the uncertainty on his face? He looked up at me, making eye contact. I raised my eyebrows as if to say, "Well, what's the verdict, Doc?" I tried desperately to read his face, instead of waiting patiently. It's not that I didn't trust him; it's just that if something was wrong, he might have run it by my mother first, and I would have had to wait. I didn't want to wait.

I wasn't sure where his inquiry was going, but I was ready for whatever it might be; probably so much more than my mother at this point. I was of age now but more importantly, I was ready for the truth. I wanted to exercise this newly acquired right to know.

I got what I asked for that day and then some. I would spend the rest of my life trying to figure out what had happened in that isolated room when all was thought lost.

It was the first time that I saw the man and not the doctor. He turned toward me, his eyes somewhat bewildered, declaring most humbly, "I don't feel anything here."

There was a brief pause then he continued, "This is quite remarkable. I know that your cancer was there before you came into the hospital, and now it isn't."

I watched this mortal god descend to ground right beside me. My first feeling was relief; actually there were two senses of relief. The obvious was that he had been unable to find any trace of the large mass that was once there; a cluster of cancerous lymph nodes. The not so obvious relief was that, up until that moment I had always seen doctors as absolute end-alls. It was the first time I felt that there were things even they didn't know for sure or couldn't fully explain, actions taking place within the body that perplexed even the professionals. It was empowering to know they might not have all things figured out. It had never occurred to me that these men and women were only human. I never thought that they too were feeling their way through life the way that I was, as we all are. This showed me there was an undeniable mystery surrounding us and not all outcomes can be predicted.

This more than evened the playing field. It gives back control to the individual where it should be, with the patient and the doctor working in unison—together.

In the doctor's mind held the knowledge of the past, in my mind, was a vision of the future. What brought us together was the present.

Proving what a great humanitarian my doctor was, he shared with me what not too many others would. It was an insight that I would never let go of. He was the one who set me on my way to chasing this mystery, with a few honest words spoken as a man. I asked him what he thought had happened.

"I think what has taken place here, David, is that you've possibly experienced some sort of spontaneous remission. Because it is so rare an occurrence, we have little understanding of it, but it does happen."

I thought. *How can cancer just go away like this?* It appeared I was smack dab in the middle of something I didn't understand. Fortunately, this was a good thing. At the time, I didn't fully grasp the significance of this. I'm not sure that I really needed to. It worked anyhow—this time—by chance.

I didn't see him for some time after, but I did take with me a precious gift, the greatest promise of all. All I had to do was find out what it was that saved me, and I had plenty of time for that. Fate would soon put me in a position to sift through the possibilities. I was about to go from one form of isolation to quite another entirely; a separation much deeper and insightful.

The last days spent at the hospital were very special to me. I was temporarily suspended between two worlds. It was a time when I was no longer in danger, so the nurses came to see me less often. When they did, there was no sense of urgency.

My appreciation for living was fierce, and my vanity had not yet entered into my consciousness. I still hadn't seen myself in the mirror to know how deeply I had been scarred. I hadn't returned home where life's routine smother's such an unusual feeling towards life. I will always remember the one particular occasion that reflected this attitude the most. My mother had come in from the outside world to see her son again, hoping to bring me home soon. Even she had gained a new optimism one can only feel when extraordinary circumstances are witnessed.

My face was riddled with the scars of chicken pox, the wound on my waist side was still fleshy but covered by bandages, and I looked vilely gaunt for a young man.

Nonetheless, I had no inhibitions—only a strong desire. It was an instant of the purest innocence one could have and still know the vanities that make us human.

I wanted so much to visit the gift store in the main lobby. I knew there were all types of magazines and souvenirs to see. I asked my mother if she would take me there. She knows me pretty well and was stunned that I didn't care what people thought. It didn't even occur to me to be conscious of the way I looked.

And don't you know? That's just what I did. Wearing just my jonnie and a pair of cheap Styrofoam slippers (standard hospital issue), I went down three floors and walked the underground tunnel to get to the main building, where I sauntered right in that little store. When people stared—which they did—sharply, I turned to them and smiled, saying "I've just had shingles." I never thought about what they might be thinking, but my mother did. I could hear her behind me adding, "He's not contagious!" I forgot to mention that part. I was excited as I looked at everything in that store as if it was the first time I had seen each thing. It was magnificent.

I was happy just to be there—to be alive. I smelled the chocolate as if someone had shoved it to my nose. The colors around me stood out as if I had just been given sight. Everything was so vivid and novel.

Mom bought me a statue of a country lad wearing a cap, sitting on the ground, enjoying a large slice of watermelon. I told her that was just the thing I was going to do when I got home. I loved watermelon.

I went back to my room and set the trophy on my rolling dinner tray. It would be the symbol of this little victory of mine that took place so far away from everything that had once brought me confidence. It would be the reminder that anything is possible. And the fact that my mother had given it to me made it that much more meaningful.

Shortly after this I went home to recover. I had lingering pain from the shingles that at times became intolerable. My mother would inject me with Demerol day and night. The summer went on this way. There was little I could do but just survive. This was a very different life for me.

I could wonder briefly, between episodes of pain, but it was hard to think about moving on. The immediate future was so imposing an impediment to seeing past it, that I had to take one day at a time. I can't explain how this felt. I held onto the promise of what I experienced. I held so tight to that hope. It was all that I had.

Fully understanding what took place in that isolation room would—for now—have to wait, although I would not forget. This knowledge of what was possible gave me something real to look forward to in the face of so much uncertainty. It was something true that surfaced after all else peeled away under the strain of a life and death struggle. It was a good feeling to know there was something greater on my side than what had tried to take my life. Now if I only knew what it was.

My desire to finally see my face in the mirror was one of the first things I realized upon my return home. I remember staring at myself, wondering who this was. My face was thin and drawn, my eyes sunken and shadowed. My skin looked like a battlefield where debris was strewn about in no particular way. The marks were freshly healing remnants of a weakening and retreating virus that left quite a mess in its wake. I tried so hard to look past this wall of reality, but at the time it devastated me. I lost so much confidence. I had survived, but it cost me dearly.

I felt so much older than my age. I was just hanging on at that point. I was not that strong young man I used to be. I was not sure that I would ever be again. What gave me confidence before was slipping away from me. The reality of what had happened was starting to sink in. I weighed about 105 lbs., down from 150 a little more than a month ago. I had been deeply scarred, emotionally and physically, by these recent events, and now I spoke faintly, with a shallow breath. I had been deflated of any airs that may have once accompanied me, posing as some sort of pride without any real foundation; pride that may have accumulated from my victories in sports. That was gone.

Nonetheless, I had to keep reminding myself that I managed the inconceivable. The one thing that keeps me looking up is the mystery that healed me when nothing else could. It provides me with so much hope; and hope gives me energy to go on. But I am still human. I still have many fears.

Where do I find the fortitude I will need to move forward when so much has been stripped from me in so little time? What will deliver me beyond my doubts when they surface? What will push me through the realm of fear to a place where true confidence will steady me, the kind of confidence which is not conditional, but a confidence that withstands? It was my sole responsibility to find this out. But where will answers come from that I can really trust enough to call my own?

Its midsummer and the humid days that define New England are spent changing dressings on my open wounds that have yet to heal after weeks of being home. I'm still receiving pain medication around the clock. My mother methodically injects me every four hours. The doctors confirm my continuing pain as residual post-herpetic neuralgia. They can't tell me when it will end. I'm tired all the time and am extremely thin. I find it difficult to eat when hurting and full of medication.

My health has reached a stalemate. I will not retreat in any way, but can't seem to get past this verge of health. I'm determined to live through this no matter what. There is so much life left to live and I plan on being there for it. I didn't go through this for nothing. On the other hand, I've been beat down enough to know not to set my sights too high. I've been disappointed before when I expect too much from myself and life. When it comes to recovery, the gains can be dreadfully slow, but if I focus and take things as they come, I can better cope with uncertainty. That's something I learned from the past that will prove to be invaluable, because what lay ahead for me could very well be my greatest trial of all.

FAR BEHIND

If I don't know how to be alone then
I am condemned to always fear loneliness.

Society glanced back briefly through its rear view mirror as my silhouette slowly diminished. I stood there speechless, motionless, as its tailwind whisked past me, sensing a profound detachment from my friends and a destiny that would never be. A part of me wanted so much to catch up, but I couldn't budge.

All of my friends had gone their separate ways. It was a time when life goals were being pursued, dreams were abundant, and well within reach—for them, that is. We were fresh out of high school, eagerly waving down taxis with diplomas in hand; the meter was ticking.

So off they went on their way to take their place in society while I withdrew into near obscurity. I'm sure none of us knew that in years to come we would look back with longing for those times. None of us appreciated the irrevocability of time. Even if we were forewarned, we probably wouldn't have listened. To us, life was endless.

I had my family to lean on, but I was finding that they were more than ready to put this behind them. That was a need I fully understood; but it just wasn't that simple for me. I felt as if I had been blindfolded, spun around violently and left to stagger as I attempted to make sense of the past, take hold of the present, and create a new life for myself.

It is a normal part of life to adjust to ever-evolving circumstances. But it's rather another thing entirely to change course completely from all that is familiar; to shed most of whom you are and begin anew.

Forging a new way requires a little more than simply putting it in the past and moving on. There was too much to be obtained by retrospection and self-examination to submit to this attitude. In the face of life and death decisions, where the stakes are their highest, there is no room for complacency or haste.

Besides, I had lived in a short time what others might not even endure in a lifetime. This was serious business as far as I was concerned. I didn't take lightly the fact that I was given a second chance to live by a force full of promise. I had squandered some precious things and moments in my past; I hoped I learned from such unnecessary losses. And if this meant embarking on the daunting task of rediscovering myself, then I was willing to do whatever it took. After all, I had nothing to lose and everything to gain. It was just as if I was starting over. I wasn't sure what to do.

I was filled with so many different thoughts and emotions. Some were evident that anyone could understand while others were hidden that only I knew of myself. I had conflicts of trust and faith, fear and courage, blame and forgiveness swirling wildly about in my mind. Many illusions of mine were about to be exposed. Most would be life changing.

I was beginning to see that there were intricate bonds leading to actions and reactions; bonds which exist on a physical, emotional, and spiritual level. They were all reliant on each other in a delicate balance of entities. And even more, such bonds tied the past to the present—intimately. The future was still free.

I began dismissing this notion that there are spontaneous occurrences when it comes to health, but rather instead—a continuum of interactions. What on the surface appeared to be a chaotic turn of events might actually have had method to its mayhem, if I could retrace this idea of cause and effect back to my actual circumstances. An empowering suggestion—that I may have played a much greater role in what eventually came to pass. This would call into question a whole way of living. If we are even somewhat instrumental in this way, then we must have much more control over our lives than we are aware of, much more than we have assumed.

A great responsibility comes with having this ability. What's more, there also comes a true freedom. This would mean that the more reactive I am in life, the more I put myself at the hands of circumstance. Conversely, the more that I am proactive—and this comes with confidence—the greater chance there is for predictable consequences and a less stressful outlook towards the near future.

So then, the way that I had perceived and interpreted, believed and reacted, in the past, had something to do with why I found myself so far from where I thought I would be at this point in my life. This detour from a proper balance within put me in a very awkward position.

This was the start of a long hard look at who I was apart from my place within my family and among my friends. I would have many opportunities to wonder about life's intentions. Complications from the therapies would plague me in the coming years, forcing me to be further separated from all that was normal. I would have to adjust to many things, many inconveniences, and it would have to be on-the-spot adaptations. I hadn't the convenience of preparation.

Those were unpredictable times. I was stuck in the realm of reactiveness. My body was feeling the repercussions of what it had been put through. There wasn't much I could do besides grin and bear it. It was like losing your paddle in the rapids and letting the currents take you as you hit and miss your way along, avoiding—simply by chance—life threatening boulders submerged underneath the shallow torrents.

It was no way to live. I would be in for many hard lessons. I was about to encounter human nature on so many levels; relations that at times made me feel proud, and at other times made me feel ashamed of myself. I didn't have the opportunity to hone my social skills in a college environment where there is some degree of tolerance should we speak or behave inappropriately. I would forego social etiquette and in its place learn just plain good manners. My transformation into adulthood would be much more hurried and crude.

The summer was the first to elude me. It was by far the hardest of all seasons to let go. After that it became easier. I let very few people into my inner circle during my recovery, probably for more than one reason; and if I'm honest with myself, I would admit that I feared how they might see me in a different way. I hadn't let go of who I used to be. That was a feat which would take some time and a lot more maturity on my part.

In the meantime, this left me alone, mostly. You could almost say that I was a stranger to myself in the beginning. I wasn't comfortable with who I saw looking back at me in the mirror. I didn't realize his strengths or see any attracting qualities that survived the onslaught of what I had been through. I was unforgiving. I hadn't the appreciation to go easy on myself. It was a very lonely experience to not love who I was. I isolated myself from others who might've showed me what I couldn't see that merited having self-worth beyond my physical abilities.

As the shingles faded by early fall I started gaining weight. It was a slow hard gain which took incredible discipline. My body was not as willing to respond to my demands. It was tired, having been through so much. Each time I pushed it, it pushed back twice as hard. Everything that I had been through was taking its toll on me.

I think the reason I focused so much on my weight was that it was tied to my strength. I couldn't gauge strength as definitively as a scale could show such physical progress.

To me, being of normal weight was a sign that I was getting better. Looking so thin and feeling so exhausted, I had trouble seeing myself as healthy. It wasn't until I was frustrated enough that I thought about the miracle that had happened, when my body nearly collapsed in isolation, and then suddenly responded. I drew from the phenomenon of that revival, a means of coping that would get me through the hardest of times thereafter.

I saw that the body heals itself; I saw it with my own two eyes. I felt it—I lived it. In no other way can a truth be as certain as having witnessed it. Even knowing this, there was a part of me that quietly longed for the past, while I lived in the ever-wavering present.

Most of my dreams were cruel to me. They would often glorify my triumphs in sports much more than they deserved to be; making me realize even more how much I had lost. In my dreams I ran with the football alongside my teammates. They were all there with me. My coaches admired me for my strength and I belonged to something greater than myself. What I did served some sort of purpose—it meant something to me. I dreamt often about my first love, that somehow time had brought her back to me. I knew that I was dreaming, even in my dreams. Fate took me so far away; I knew that there was no going back. Sometimes it seemed so real to me that my heart would ache right after and I would feel again the full extent of my losses as if they had just happened.

This became a defining theme that in the early years would haunt me until I came to terms with acceptance and this idea of loss and gain as part of living life. Many conceptions that I once held would eventually succumb to this new reality.

My belief in fairness for instance would be one of the first casualties of this transformation. Fairness in life is relative, subjective, assumptive and bordering on the naïve. Tradition might very well be to blame for this array of confusion. What I have found is that there are tendencies for life to be justified—conditional tendencies. In other words, life is fundamentally impartial, but it tends towards evenhandedness and order, both of which can have very unpleasant outcomes.

Not to say that life isn't random—it is, but there are an infinite amount of conditions around us that influence its path; conditions that humanity may be directly or indirectly responsible for. It can be complicated. That's why it may seem that life lives up to its alter-reputation of having malice, of being callous and condemnatory.

How we look at life makes a big difference in the way that we deal with it. Why things happen isn't always so easily seen by the naked eye. I would say that most of what occurs in life may not be readily understandable, but is definitively traceable. Actions will always have an origin.

I needed to know that there was no hidden hand in my fate. It meant a lot to me that I was not just living some preset destiny. That would not have made much sense to me. If I was free, then I would take this notion for everything it was worth, in every aspect of my life. That's how I would want it.

The years that followed would prove this to me intimately. They would clearly show me that I was responsible, that we all are to a certain extent, responsible for our conditions. And if we aren't responsible on a personal level, than collectively we bear some liability for what happens to the individual.

I know that this is not a popular explanation. It's much harder to accept; but this way of thought allowed me to better handle what I could and couldn't change. It empowered me. It drew attention to the present and put the past in its place rather than allowing unresolved feelings of guilt and an inability to forgive myself for actions beyond my control, yet caused by me, to get in the way. It was the kind of guilt that wore down my defenses just as effectively as the manifestation of cancer did.

Just three months before being diagnosed with Hodgkin's disease, I was involved in an accident with my best friend, Dean. We were high school buddies, just starting off in life with every bit of orneriness one would imagine of sixteen-year-olds just given their freedom to drive. These were adventurous times and we both did all that we could to make the most of them. Our sophomore year had ended and the first summer with our cars was upon us. We cut loose.

Sultry days were spent on the shorelines of Newport, Scarborough, Narragansett, Matunuck, and Beavertail in Jamestown. And if we had enough money for gas, we'd venture to Misquamicut, where the riptides were most robust. We roamed the beaches like wandering gypsies, waking up on the sands after a wild evening in the local nightspots. It was good clean fun though; no one got hurt. We'd crash beach-house parties after hearing about them while body-surfing the waves for hours. No one we knew, but that's what made it so exciting. I don't think we ever got much rest then—not that we needed it. At that moment in time the world was ours.

Then one day came—it came to us like rolling thunder. It was midsummer; we were that much closer to our junior year. The rain fell out of the sky heavy and ominous, drowning any thought of driving to the coastlines like we'd done for so many days before. We caught a movie instead, just to do something. We were almost home—less than a mile or so. The road split directions; turning right would've taken us to my house, and left—to Dean's, by way of a notorious winding road.

I asked Dean if he wanted to hang out at my house for a while until the rain let up, but he promised his mother he'd be back to watch his sisters while she went to work. With that, I headed left, down that winding road, as the rain pelted the windshield. I was driving the limit which was no more than twenty-five or thirty miles per hour. The curves were tight—very tight.

About halfway down, I drove right through a large puddle of water. I lost the steering as the electrical system failed. It had shorted out from the surge of water underneath the carriage. The wheel would not negotiate. At that point we both became passengers, while chance grabbed the wheel from me. The car hydroplaned wildly across the street—right towards a massive oak tree. It happened in a split second. There was no time to react or brace ourselves. There was a loud crash—then silence. There was no skidding or screeching noises to be heard, just the impact itself, and the sound of crushing metal. The steering wheel hit my chest and bent in half. Dean wasn't as lucky. His head hit the dashboard. He went out right away. It was the most sickening feeling to see my best friend's head slam the dashboard on impact. There was nothing I could do to save him from this.

It was so quiet after. He laid there unconscious. I was in shock. The only thing that jolted me to act was seeing the engine ignite in flames after the hood had crushed open from the blow. I called to my buddy over and over. I didn't know if he was dead or not. So much emotion raced through me. I jumped from the car and ran around to his side. The door had trouble opening but it finally gave way. I grabbed hold of Dean—anywhere I was able to get a decent grip, and pulled him from the vehicle. I then dragged him far enough away from the danger. In a panic, I left him to find someone around that could help us. I nearly broke a stranger's door down as I frantically yelled for assistance. Then at last, a woman answered and immediately called emergency. I don't remember much of what followed, except being in the emergency room a short time after.

Dean was admitted to Rhode Island Hospital in critical condition, where he remained in a semi-coma for fourteen days. It was by far the worst time of my life. Those days were devastating. I wanted him to wake. Every day he slept, some life in me slowly slipped away. What I didn't know then was that he lay in the very place where I too would be destined to fight for my life. It was just a matter of time before his theatre would become mine.

I blamed myself for what happened to my best friend because I was driving. All that I remember was being entangled in a dangerous web of guilt. I always felt things deeply, a character trait that can be at times a double edged sword.

My friend finally regained consciousness, but he was never fully the same. Those closest to him could really tell the difference. All of his recent memories were gone. Unfortunately I was part of those memories. I kept waiting for him to remember—most of all, to remember me, but he barely knew me, or all the times we shared together.

So much had changed in so short a time. It was the end of an era of innocence and infallibility.

I tried the best way I knew to bond with Dean again, but it would never be what it had been. I realized then how life can change with such permanence. Time and my falling ill became the wedge between us, until at last our friendship had all but succumbed. Reluctantly, I let go of him, and then the thought of him; eventually, we went our separate ways.

I took away from this a deep sense of guilt. I bore it as if I could get away with such a heavy burden. I never forgave myself or really ever knew how, nor was anyone there to explain how these things happen in life and sometimes no one is to blame. I figured my best friend was hurt and someone had to answer for that, and that someone was me. I pushed the guilt deep down inside until I didn't think about it every single day after. But I was fooling myself. It was always there—simmering—like venomous poison. Instead of releasing the guilt, and somehow working it out in my mind, I owned every bit of it; it smothered me.

I went into my junior year carrying this emotional baggage as one would his books or a back pack. I went without my best friend. It was surreal. I was there but I really wasn't.

He was still home recovering. I didn't play football that year. What I didn't know was that I would never compete in this way, ever again. The guilt I felt made me vulnerable to illness. Three months after the accident I was diagnosed with cancer—Hodgkin's Disease, to be specific; a type of autoimmune disease in which the body attacks itself.

Was this coincidence? I say no. It was probably more a result of the manifestation of my destructive thoughts and emotions. I punished myself for the accident.

It wasn't until I started to look back that it made sense to me; especially in light of my ensuing discoveries.

So how did knowing this help me through? It did, in so many ways. I was able to look at cancer in context rather than perceiving it as mysterious and unapproachable. I could begin to know my enemy by knowing its habits—if you will. Cancer then becomes traceable, and dare I say—almost predictable. Not always. Life doesn't work that way. If we trace the evidence of this elusive force—circumstantially, that is, trace it in terms of indirect markers, whether they be physical or psychological, then we don't need to actually define cancer to defend ourselves from it, but rather understand the cause and effect of its presence through looking at these physical and emotional markers, naturally pointing to a possible imbalance within us. If they are evident, then we begin to connect the dots. This demystifies; this brings clarity.

I didn't really need to know about cancer so much as I needed to know what I could do to better protect myself from it. That was the extent of my interest. I was never obsessed with the disease itself. I saw no reason to be. Besides, there were so many complications to deal with after the therapies that I had no time to really think about cancer or whether it would return again. I had no such fear or hunch. I trusted what had healed me.

I did see however, the role I played in allowing the proper environment for it to come about. There is a monumental difference.

There were new obstacles and threats to my health that more than deserved my attention.

Most complications that I weathered were opportunistic. My immune system was impaired. I had no spleen to ward off certain dangerous bacterial infections. My lungs had just been bombarded with radiation so they were compromised as well. This set the stage for pneumonia—both bacterial and viral; walking pneumonia as well. And I had another similar bout with the same bacterial blood infection that I contracted in isolation. It was a very frightening thing. I never knew what to expect. It happened so spontaneously.

I went to bed one night feeling no different than any other night. I woke sometime later lying in sweat—the sheets drenched. I sweltered. I got up fast, sensing I was in the middle of something I didn't understand, but yet knew enough to do something about it—immediately. I yelled for someone; my mother followed me to the bathroom where I had instinctively sought cold water. I couldn't get there fast enough. Before I reached the sink I passed out and slammed my head against the tile floor. I came to after hearing the sounds of my mother's voice pleading with me to explain what was happening. She was petrified. There was no time to answer her; at this point I was acting on pure instinct. I managed to grab the sink from the floor and pulled myself up enough to turn the water on. I began cupping the water and violently splashing it to my face. I was calling to her, "Water mom, water!"

She ran for the phone and dialed for help. I could hear the sirens blaring throughout the early morning hours, until they were right in front of our house. I left almost immediately on a stretcher—layered in linen, wrapped in a cocoon. I couldn't answer the paramedic's questions because I was shivering uncontrollably; my teeth chattered as well.

I spent the next couple of weeks on IV antibiotics while my weight plummeted once again to near emaciation.

When pneumonia struck it really set me back. I lost precious weight and was fatigued for many weeks after returning home from being in the hospital for so long.

While in the hospital, I would have physical therapists come into my room to tap on my chest and back, in an effort to help clear my lungs and keep them from further congesting. Between these attacks on my immune system, I would have periodic episodes of radiation enteritis to deal with. I spent so much time in the emergency room for this condition alone that the doctors and nurses began to remember me.

It was a notably large emergency room with many stalls and a continually rotating staff. I don't remember making too much of an impression, in fact, I did more observing than anything else. I was always a quiet patient. I was humbled by this profession. I respected it.

That is not to say that I wasn't assertive when the situation called for it. As I began to realize how important it was to be aware of human error, I started to pay close attention to procedures done on me. There were times I kept them sharp and on their toes. I made sure they thought about things when I noticed routine was setting in. This was done gently and usually without them ever realizing their proficiency had just been called out. You never get anywhere bruising an ego or whittling away at someone's self-esteem. That was something I didn't have to learn the hard way; I just knew it. That said, it was a rare event that I would need to speak up; usually everything was done well.

I gained most of my respect for the medical profession—at Rhode Island Hospital. It became my home away from home. It is also where I learned so much about people in general. I picked up certain social skills while in the company of remarkably talented men and women. It was there I came to know some common virtues which shaped my character in the midst of fighting for my life; virtues that sometimes take a good dose of humility to help assimilate. What comes to mind are two of the most impressionable instances of learning the hard way that I can readily remember—detail to detail.

On one occasion, I was placed in a four-person room during an episode of enteritis. Directly across from me was a black man of middle age. He appeared unkempt. It was the first thing that I noticed. Then I was drawn to his eyes. They seemed troubled and shifty—but sincere. He looked terribly uncomfortable. I often caught him looking my way with a more than just a curious stare. I felt he was trying to kindle a conversation. Exchanging words might've sidetracked his pain if I had indulged him, but I wasn't the kind for small talk. I was private when in the hospital and unless the exchange went somewhere, I preferred to abstain. I was getting used to hearing other patients whine about the small stuff. I would rather it had to do with something besides noting how the nurses seldom answered the buzzer right away or how the hospital food wasn't like home cooking. I realized from having a mother in the profession, how overwhelmed a nurse can be when he or she is delegated more and more responsibility. My mother came home so tired at the end of her shift. I respected that dedication. To me the nurse was not a servant but a caregiver. I know that it takes a very special person to become a nurse; I know that person would have to really care for people in a way that rises above the rest of us. That person has compassion so deeply seated in their character that no amount of foul smell, bed sores, difficult patients, hard to find veins, cleaning of urine or crap in a bed, could ever change their devotion to the sick. That's who they are. My mother did this in a state hospital for decades before retiring. How can I measure her any other way than to say that she had God in her? How can we measure any of them any other way? Of course they're human—we all are. So when it comes to them being at times cranky or not rushing to the patients every whim, for me—they get a pass.

This was different. I could see that he had no intention of complaining. I guess I should've given this man a chance before dismissing him. It wasn't fair. I had been in and out of that hospital so much that sometimes I just wanted to get through with it alone.

Whether I wanted to or not he was determined to have some sort of dialogue with me. I admire determination; even if it imposes on me. I took a different view by now, of him.

His face distorted as he mumbled at me, quick, jaggedly and with a low, almost inaudible voice. I could barely hear him—I leaned towards him while straining to listen. I may not have wanted this, but I was never raised to be disrespectful.

I thought I heard him trying to say that he was hurting badly. I could tell that he was extremely restless. He was a stranger to me, more than just not knowing him. This was a man of a different race that I had had very little interaction with in my life. I was unsure how to relate with him. I didn't want to offend him in any way.

He couldn't seem to get comfortable. He kept reaching towards his back. I gathered this was the problem. When I asked him what he needed, he said that the pain medication was not working, that what he was getting wasn't enough. I'm ashamed to say this but given the initial impression I had of him, I thought he might want drugs for other reasons, and this was his way of getting them. I held this opinion with little conviction—but held it. I told him that if it hurt enough he should speak up and let the doctors know. He seemed somewhat animated and quite dramatic.

The days went by as I listened in on his discussions with the hospital staff. I noticed his care lacked the personal emotional touch that one would expect, given his condition.

After several days I finally saw his family. It was his mother and sisters. They were gentle people and polite towards me. I remember how they cared for him, this scruffy soul who looked like he spent most of the time living hard and possibly without the basic amenities.

The next morning the house doctor visited as usual, accompanied by his staff. But this time he brought with him grave news. Nineteen years later I can tell you word for word what was said, simply because of the impression it made on me. The conversation was basically one-sided as the man listened to his sentence. The doctor told him that his tests showed a large tumor wrapped tightly around his spine, the place where I had often seen him grab for while wincing. The doctor also acknowledged his need for more medication and said he would immediately up the dosage. He—in his own way—which I thought was done compassionately, explained that the situation was terminal and promised to do everything in his power to keep him comfortable. Then he left the room.

By now the man realized that we had both shared his news. His eyes widened. I didn't know what to say so I remained still, but I didn't look away from him. I felt ashamed of myself for judging him. I felt it so strongly that I thought he could almost feel my guilt from across the room.

I didn't know how to react. There was nothing I could've said to change what he had just heard—nothing. No one can teach you these things the way experience does. No amount of schooling can instill such raw truth into one's being. Nothing but moments like these has the ability to bring character-altering feelings—like humiliation and shame—to one's awareness. To see that this man had days if not weeks to live, to see this firsthand, affected me. I felt immense compassion for him and I thank God he couldn't see through my guise straight to my ignorance.

No response would've been appropriate; at least that much I got right. I kept my mouth shut and thought about what I fool I'd been. The nurse came right in afterwards with an effective dose of medicine. This saved me. I could see that it helped him. There were no signs of suffering thereafter. His face relaxed—so did I.

I was discharged from the hospital before I knew what became of him. It was the middle of the winter; the winds were unforgivingly cold, and the air uncomfortably raw.

I thought about him a lot when I was home. I couldn't get him out of my mind. I really wanted to know what he was going through. I felt a human bond with him on a level I didn't understand then. But in some way I wanted to calm him or at the very least, reach out to show I cared. I wanted to be more to him than I was. I felt that call; it was a strong one. I tried to talk myself out of it. I asked myself: *I didn't really know him, so why did I care? What difference was I going to make?*

The truth was I did care. I felt an urge to make things right between us. I really thought it made a difference. On some level I couldn't explain then, I needed to do these things.

After a week of hesitation I decided to visit him, driving into the city at night. I brought with me snacks I remembered he craved so much. He said that when he got home the first thing he would eat were Oreos, peanut butter and Snickers. It wasn't much to offer. I couldn't give him his life back, or more days to live, but this gesture might show him that he made a difference in someone's life; it might show him that I cared.

When I arrived I didn't find him in the room. I expected the worst. I went to the nurse's station and asked about him. They had moved him onto another floor.

I was relieved. When I got near the door of his room I could see that he was now in a private room. This was good. This was how it should be. It was proper.

I wasn't sure what to expect, so when I entered I was pleased to see him still aware and with his family close to his bed. They were grateful to see me and thanked me for thinking about him. I could see that he was in much more pain than before. Things had gotten much worse. I handed him my offering and he gratefully accepted with a smile.

I didn't stay very long but I did feel so much better than if I'd stayed home and only wished I had come.

Another week had passed and my concern got the best of me. I made another trip to the city to see him again. This time was much different, as the mood of the room had changed dramatically; no longer were there smiles to greet me. Death was in the air. His family was again there by his side, but I didn't recognize the man in the bed. He was unaware of anyone in his room and not with peace at all. Fear had filled his eyes with a cold unattached stare as he thrashed up and down in a most desperate way.

I knew I had walked in on a private moment not meant for anybody but loved ones. I'll never forget the feeling I got when I saw him so at odds with his own death, so scared. He wasn't ready to die; not like this. I don't know what was going through his mind but I thought death shouldn't be this way. It shouldn't come to us so completely unannounced. There was something so unnatural about it.

I never saw him again; although he's never left me. I'm reminded of him every time I begin to judge anyone on preconceptions. The thought of him keeps me just. Life was watching me; it pays close attention when such moments define character. I hope I didn't let it down.

Few occasions stand out enough to declare that we're different people because of them. That was one—this situation would be another.

Again, I was placed in a four-person room. I don't recall the reason for being admitted, just the fact that I was there again. The men around me were all much older. It was a theme I was used to. The oldest patient by far was lying diagonally across from me. He was unconscious most of the time but managed to moan and groan incessantly throughout the night. He did a very good job of keeping some of us awake, not only in our room but in the nearby stalls. I had been there a few days and it was starting to wear on me. I couldn't sleep well and I really needed to get some rest.

It was around two or three in the morning. I was awakened again by the moans. They were long, drawn out and loud. Eventually I became annoyed enough to silently wish him to shut up, anything to make him stop the noise so that I could fall back asleep. I stared his way, just watching him, wondering when the heck it would end. He took deep labored breaths, mesmerizing me. I paid close attention to each and every inhale and exhale of his. I didn't think about what was making him this way. He was very old and tired.

Just as his breathing brought me into a hypnotic, rhythmic state—on the exhale, it suddenly stopped. The unexpected change in pace startled me into attention. I stared now, intently, at his chest. There was nothing, just stillness. Could it be that I was watching a man die right in front of me?

When I was certain he was no longer breathing I pressed the button for the nurse. She responded immediately; she asked me if everything was alright.

Through the shaded room, I pointed across to the elderly man, saying, "I think he stopped breathing." She called a code blue. Within minutes the room was filled with emergency staff trying to resuscitate the gentleman. It was something to see, this trueness of the moment. My eyes welled up as I looked on with sadness and shame.

I felt terrible about the way I'd carried on in my mind. *They had to revive him.* I hoped.

It took some time for him to be stabilized but they were finally able to accomplish this. I realized that if I hadn't been watching him at that crazy hour in the night, he would certainly have passed away.

As quickly as they filled the room, they were gone and I was left with him alone. Yes, there were two other patients in the beds next to us, but they were out of it; both their curtains were drawn. I looked over to this old man who was given another chance, and an immense feeling overcame me. I got out of bed and walked towards him as he lay there silent for the moment—almost peaceful. As I got closer to the bed I saw a large figure of a man. He was much more real to me as I stood above him, next to him. His hands were massive, very much like my great grandfather's, who toiled right until his death. This was a once strong and able being who lay there near the end of his life, full of memories that only he will ever know. He was loved by someone at some time. He had stories to be told that would never be.

As his giant hand hung off the side of the bed, I took hold of it. Grasping to it, I told him how sorry I was to have been so selfish. I asked him to forgive me and that I would never be so insensitive again. I'm sure that he didn't hear a word of this, but I know some-how—someone or something beside me was there to bear witness. Something wonderful was in that room to make things right, to clear the air between two people.

There were other virtues worthy of mention that I learned as a result of my experiences in and out of the hospital. I learned patience when my body was taking its time to heal, determination to see my way through in the face of physical and emotional exhaustion, and moderation of medicines that were given to me for pain, to use at my judgment. I learned to trust and to be trusted. I learned the art of simplicity; using words with direction and clarity to best describe my symptoms, to be understood in the environment of my care.

I became flexible to change in situations beyond my control; when my blood work had to be drawn at four-thirty in the morning or sometimes even earlier, or when personnel in transport would unexpectedly come into my room during lunch or dinner to take me for an X-ray, ultrasound, or CT scan, or just as my family had arrived to visit me, or when I was so tired I would rather have gone to sleep. And of course I learned to be responsible for myself, to be alert at all times for changes in my body; whether they be reactions from medications or subtle symptoms overlooked by a doctor or a nurse. I realized that it was my life. No one would care for it more than me. No one should care for it more than me.

It would be easy to say theoretically that the professionals are there to see to your recovery; that it's their job to make sure everything goes right while you're under their care. In a perfect world that thought would be half true—at best. But we don't live in a perfect world; life seldom follows theory. In this life—shit happens. And when it's my life at stake, passing the responsibility baton to someone else is a risk I'm not willing to take. It's just not good sense. I can both admire and respect medical professionals and at the same time know that they are people too—people make mistakes. There's no good and bad here—it's not about that at all. It's about prudence. That's really all it's about—living responsibly.

I think more than anything else, what I came away with from my interactions with other patients, doctors and nurses was that I was beginning to know myself and what life expected of me. I was realizing this person who went through a terrible ordeal and changed so much because of it.

I was discovering new strengths, while letting go of tired, worn-out perceptions, and liking what I saw in the mirror once again. An entirely different human being was emerging from the ashes of a broken one. I was learning how life rejuvenates even the most fatigued of us.

I was gaining a deeper confidence that was not conditional upon physical strength or how others perceived me; a confidence that was not based on my ego, which can be very unsteady, but instead reliant on a force much greater than me, a force that flows through us—healing us. I found new confidence which showed me how—through hardships—the body does recuperate and can become even stronger.

I also had the confidence of familiarity. I was exposed to my fears again and again, finally seeing them for what they were—mostly just conceptual fears.

And then there was the unexpected confidence that I inherited from bringing comfort to others who shared their personal concerns with me. To them, I said what I felt. I believed what I told them because I had lived it. They could see this passion in me; they could see that I was serious when I said that they would be all right. I would tell them not to worry, that they would find the strength to overcome. It would be there for them. To me those weren't just words.

When I said these things, I meant it and they knew it. When I didn't mean it or feel it, I said nothing. I saw in their eyes—trust in this.

Then they would look at me—smile—and thank me; they would thank me. I couldn't believe it. I wanted to thank them for letting me into their world. I needed them as much as they may have needed me, probably a bit more. What gave me this confidence to empower them—I couldn't say; it just came natural to me. But more than anything else, it made a difference in their outlook. I was beginning to discover qualities of my character through these very relations. I began to feel good about myself and the small contributions I offered whenever I had the chance. They had worth—which meant I had worth.

Still, I was a long way from home. I felt a great sense of separation from others that at times saddened me. Who I was, my many complications, the unfortunate stigma of where I'd been, not yet knowing where I fit in, were all things which further separated me from a true bond with others. I still had no idea how to get back or where my place in society would be.

I was gaining more confidence in life—true confidence; confidence that survives a direct blow to vanity, confidence that makes me more than just myself, but part of a greater calling that gives me a selfless strength—a just strength. This sustains.

But it still meant nothing to me if I couldn't share this insight to empower others.

While I was finding my true self I had inadvertently lost my way. I was no longer that person who held a certain place. The road back, if there was one at all, had yet to be revealed.

I lived with this detachment for many years. Physical, emotional, and spiritual boundaries all kept me just out of reach. I had no choice than to get to know who I was and who I wasn't. How could I know about life if I didn't know who I was or what was important? If I was going to learn how not to be lonely than I must really learn what it meant to be alone. In order to love others in a way that means something more than words, I had to begin to love myself in a way that forgave my faults and weaknesses, in a way that nourished my virtues and brought out the best in me. Maybe then I wouldn't have to search for that indefinable home that would lend me meaning and purpose; maybe it just might find me.

LIFE UNDER
PROVIDENCE

I've heard how there is a reason for everything that happens; I've heard this throughout my lifetime. The echoes of this thought surface again and again like some infallible, eternal verity. Simple words said, so often without thought, yet behind them is so much meaning.

What compels some to think beyond these words—to the truth of them, while so many others are satisfied with the surface meaning? Is it enough simply to hear that everything happens for a reason? Will believing this without grounds actually empower us? There are matters in life worth more careful consideration; life under providence will lead us to their discovery.

Rather than saying that things happen for a reason, I would agree more with the law of cause and effect. This is more definable and much less vague a notion. It tells us that there are reactions to actions, which make our lives self-sanctioning, when we understand that every action of ours will bring a response of some sort. Each and every action and reaction holds the potential to take us in a certain direction in life. Either we are an imposing force in our own destiny, which means that we know who we are, what we are here for, what we want in life, what our strengths are, and where we are going, or we are reacting to the many influences that assail us throughout life, and therefore are left dangerously at the whim of circumstance—a destiny of reactions to outward influence.

If ever there was a lasting certainty that no span of time could deny, it would have to be the assurance that life actively seeks a way to live through any threat which tests its determination to survive. The fact that I have made it this far in my life has less to do with chance and more to do with never giving up. It's clear to me that while chance may bring to your doorstep opportunity, it is not as a rule what saves you from the forces that destroy.

There are certain attributes that almost always define a true survivor, and one is never without all of them at any given time. We hear these stories over and over about heroic survival against all odds and wonder in awe, but our first instinct is to separate ourselves from these miracles, to put them above reach. For some reason we place an unseen barrier between our understanding of them and their promise. We separate ourselves by thinking that there was something different about that person who experienced this phenomena; something we don't have. We say to ourselves that we are not that fortunate. Some may even think that it was a blessing and silently declare that they don't deserve to be blessed.

These are self-defeating attitudes, and are the ways in which we turn from the healing force, which is an everlasting energy meant for every one of us. Every one of us! If I were to try and explain what it is about me that's most determined to resist succumbing in any way, I would have to say that I have seen past many of the distractions in life—right through to the truth of death. Even more, I've listened to those nearest to dying, because they are holding the secret of the ages. The passion which eludes so many of the living seems not to escape those at the threshold of life and death. They are struggling for their every breath taken, hoping to see another tomorrow, and seeing things very few are able to. If you listen to them as if your life depended on it, you would come away with so much more appreciation for life. I have heard these words clearly; I've seen their expressions. I could never misinterpret what they are conveying. It is so clear.

"Fight, fight hard for your life!" They cry out to me. "Fight with everything you have inside, and let no end come without a full and honest engagement of all your senses. Search around you for the most inspiring beauty and fill your eyes with such, until they overflow with color and shades of the brightest and most vivid earth-tones. Smell—if even a hint, the fragrance of the youth; it is nearest to life. Welcome the taste of the tart and the bitter—the sweet will be that much sweeter on your tongue. Hear the perfection of the chords of nature's symphony from out of your window. Touch ever so gently, the ones you love; feel their affection for you. And lastly, sense what others cannot begin to know—that a mystery envelopes you; it protects you.

Say not farewell. For if you have the strength to utter such words, than you are not ready to die, and what you have left must fight on!"

So how do we do this? How do we reach this deep into a reservoir that we are—at the very most—vaguely familiar with? What part of us rises to such an occasion, to such heights, after we've exhausted our bodies and have so little energy left to go on? If it's not something I can touch or see, like my physical self, then how can it be real or effective? How can it help me in this tangible world that I live in where the five senses is all I've ever really known? What promise of life guides my spirit through the very struggle between life and death? What will lend any of us the strength to bear pain and overcome suffering, despair, loneliness, sorrow and loss?

These are the fundamental questions haunting us since creative thought began. There is very good reason for this. From the moment in our past that we freed ourselves from the instinctual mind, that is, from the time we realized our ability to choose, to be aware, we've assumed the responsibility of our destiny in very serious, dynamic ways. This evolution of thought has its origins in the higher laws of life. We must recognize this in order to keep the balance among the inward and outward relating entities.

Since spontaneously recovering from a near death experience, I've been left with the fallout of these questions that I must come to understand on my own in order for me to be truly prepared for life's rude den should it ever insist on my entering it again. I've been given a second chance in life, and because of this I must know next time the place where I can look to when medicine reaches its limits. The miracle I've heard about while I was young and felt personally, in my teens, is familiar to me now—attainable, like never before. I will never forget what I've learned about life's promise. This is what held my attention in the years that followed my immediate recovery.

There was isolation like I had known while in the hospital, but I never expected that when I returned home I would experience a deeper, more profound isolation that would alter everything about me. As much as I initially felt at odds being alone, I began to welcome it almost defiantly. In my mind I would never let my circumstance get the best of me. I adapted to whatever was thrown at me; I adapted on purpose. A part of me desperately resisted this stranger that I was to myself, while another part of me knew that somewhere in this unknown lay the answers to many of my deepest concerns. I would have to live through the loneliness until I was no longer lonely but simply alone, and eventually at ease with this feeling. At first, in my mind, I kicked and screamed and wanted nothing to do with this solitude; an effort that could prevent me from knowing my true self, instead of the one cast by society's form. It took a little time to break the habit of being distracted, but my mind was creative enough and my will stoic enough to overcome this deficit.

In doing so, day after day I felt more comfortable with the unfamiliar, more comfortable with myself. Time passed in the way of weeks and months without my noticing it, when I began to realize that I was not alone at all but in the company of myself and all of humanity as well; after which I was no longer uneasy. I was also beginning to feel a sense of freedom on my own because I had been freed from the restraints of distraction and influence. The fear of being alone was no longer gnawing at my spirit. Eventually, I was left in harmony with aloneness because I was beginning to forgive my past; I was beginning the long journey of knowing myself and respecting my freshly formed qualities.

Life might make us weather periods of isolation; that is not as important as how we handle it and that we use this separation to our advantage. I will testify to the edifying effects of being in my own company, without any diversions. It is very easy to get sidetracked due to the pressures of everyday life, which seem to have a way of intruding into one's attention. So I knew from early on that in order to stay with this gift of awareness I would have to live under Providence. I would have to be vigilant about what deserves my attention. I would have to realize the things in life that are most important to survival; not just mine but others' as well. These were the only things I would invest my attention in.

There are laws of nature that are adhered to by the living world, all of which are instinctive and as such—involuntary. Humanity however, is a privileged species in that we have, somewhere along the evolutionary timeline, liberated ourselves from this instinctual bond with nature. In doing so, our minds have evolved according to this fairly newfound freedom. In evolutionary measurements, this liberation, or self-awareness, is brief in regards to life's history. So we've just begun to realize our potential with this newly acquired entity of our mind—I call the creative mind, which is an evolving part of the mind that at some point became aware of its existence and moved away from instinct. It is the one entity that has the ability and will to create a new way from the old. It has freed itself from the inherent mind, and then eventually evolved enough to guide and govern it.

The creative mind is of a voluntary nature, and puts us above all other living things that are without the virtues of higher laws.

Sometimes I feel, while considering our violent and greed filled history that we have been negligent, that humanity wasn't yet prepared to go it alone. Our maturity did not evolve hand in hand with our rebellious need to do our own thing. Nonetheless, humanity is already on its way. We have a lot of catching up to do, and we have to start somewhere.

So what have we done with this freedom of the mind, this liberation from fate? What guides us now that we have choice and are no longer slaves to an instinctual rule of law, where nature dictates our actions in every aspect of life—or mere survival? How does this affect our wellbeing, that is, to have a thinking mind which discerns? Through this evolution, we have greatly empowered ourselves. In comparison though, I would say that we are like infants wielding a loaded weapon.

With this empowerment brings an even greater responsibility to each other, and the more vulnerable—animal kingdom. This responsibility includes proper perception and interpretation of one's circumstances. Perception is the way we look at what happens to us and around us, and that understanding may be somewhat skewed if we're perceiving things through the guise of preconceived notions, beliefs, judgments and even self-defeating attitudes. All are a part of our recent and distant history, which leaves an impression upon the mind that may or may not be indelible, depending upon how we interpret such. In that interpretation contains the seeds of response, which leads to an array of emotional reactions that we already know influence the immune system by way of the central nervous system. This self-empowerment has the potential to be very helpful; but if there is no responsibility attached with it, no understanding of this, then this same privilege can also be very destructive, with repercussions felt, such as disease. This is in no way a leap of deduction, because I have, more or less, taken you to this understanding in progressive steps. I have lived through this understanding myself, slowly, methodically.

I saw that responsibility had become a prevailing theme throughout notions of self-empowerment. I realized that having a sense of freedom also meant that there must be rules to live by. Freedom has conditions that cannot be separated.

As far as living with the intelligence of the life force, which has the capacity to rejuvenate, a choice must be made to listen to that which only the individual can come to know on one's own. These truths are higher laws.

The way that I perceive life, then, becomes my reality. This can happen without me really noticing the actual distance between my interpretation of truth and what really is. How do we let our thoughts and emotions twist and distort our vision to such a degree that it leaves us vulnerable to the great higher laws of life? If I begin to unravel the answer to this dilemma, which I believe is the single most important impediment to closing the gap between how I see things instead of the way they really are, then I will be that much closer to understanding the mystery of the vital life force—that much closer to confidence. And when I have confidence I am without fear, doubt and hesitation. I am no longer vulnerable, but indeed—empowered and imposing, all while living under providence.

DELIVERANCE

Evolution does not fly in the face of God...
the essence of God takes flight in evolution.

Everything that lives—evolves; nothing remains the same.
I could not remain the same person I was. I finally realized this. Therefore, an idea of religion that I have grown up with hung dangling in the balance of a spirituality in transition—my spirituality. Through what I have lived and because of what I have come to know, I was no longer in the same place. What I thought would never happen—happened; I lost my religion. I'm not sure it was really mine to begin with. But that did not make it any easier. Letting go of something that you've leaned on for most of your life should never be taken lightly. Our shared religion was a common thread that helped bond our family through uncertain times. It gave us hope.

I know that my mother bore it the hardest. She would never tell me, but I could see it in her eyes many times when the subject happened to come up. If I regretted anything it would be that she had seen this separation in me. It wasn't something I could hide for very long in a family so close, with a mother so close. I never meant to hurt her. I wasn't concerned what anyone else thought because it was my life. But my mother was everything to me; she deserved so much from her son. I felt that I had disappointed her.

This new life that I was forging required that I be true to myself, that I know intimately what moves me. There could be no doubts, hesitation, or conveniences; my convictions had to be my own. I knew that my mother would understand this in time. I knew that her emotions would settle and she would eventually see that I was an individual in discovery. It's one of the reasons why I love her so much. My mother considered these things.

The answers had not come to me; they were not there for me. I wasn't able to replace what had been lost with another belief. It was not like that. But this wasn't a reason to turn back. I was out there— on my own now, and I was all right.

I held on to promises that I had witnessed personally. I couldn't explain them right away, but I knew they were real and very relevant in my life. I also knew that they were powerfully influential; influential enough to bring me this kind of confidence. At the time, it was all that I needed to know. There was something about what I was in touch with that made me feel comfortable going it alone. I was back to basics, back to building a foundation that I could stand on, only this time I would be the one to build it.

I was evolving through this hardship, because of this hardship. Of all that has changed in my life, this has the most; it has also been the hardest for me to do. Anyone could see the superficial changes as I went through what I did; even a stranger could see that I had been affected by something unusual. Some of these changes were obvious, but so much more was taking place within me. It was a revolution of discoveries and realizations, some having had much deeper roots than others.

It's not easy to live through the life-threatening circumstances that brought me to the brink of death and still remain the same person. That's impossible. As a result, there was a certain truth that I demanded of life—actually, that life demanded of me, and I would do whatever it would take to live by it. You could say at this point that I was being guided from within. That would be true.

Maybe I felt this way many years ago when I was still young, which could be why I explored life so passionately while growing up. Maybe my rebellious ways held within them hints of this desire to know myself in this way, to know life in this way, to be closer to the truth.

Some might say that I was asking too much of myself; in a way, they would be right. But I would rather ask too much of myself than settle for too little. This high road I sought was a hard road.

I lost my way during the years that followed my stay in isolation. It was a trying time for me. I put myself through so much. I pushed myself hard, physically and emotionally. My spirituality remained undefined. There was an imbalance in my life because of this. Still I searched.

I was torn between the past and my present, knowing I couldn't live in two worlds, yet not knowing how to escape the past or at least how to separate the two. I was frustrated with myself for not knowing what to do, but not enough to ask for counsel.

Feelings of promise and hope stayed with me; these inspirations followed me where no one could.

There was a mystery that I knew was there but I was a long way away from knowing it with any certainty. I felt its presence. It gave me confidence as well as peace of mind at times when I needed it the most. This feeling stayed with me—never letting me experience loneliness, even when it loomed about me.

I wondered if my seeing things differently would possibly open the door to another way through life. I have always felt religious; the way of life inspires me. But it had to be my own religion. It had to be something that I felt from my heart.

My search for truth had a greater hold on me since recovering from cancer. And I saw the importance of believing things of this nature with all of my being. I once had blind faith and it didn't protect me. I once thought the doctors were like gods—they weren't. I once thought the world was just—another belief of mine that had been exposed.

It was time to be confident and sure of what I believed. There could be no room for doubt with something so close to the inner core of who I was. Even though my past was filled with tradition and religion, it wasn't enough to settle me, and yet I could not get away from the feeling that there was something there—beyond the rituals, sermons, and congregation.

There was something about the way we needed each other. There was a part of me that hungered for this bond to others. It was real. It was something I would never let go of.

And a truth survived through all the confusion. It was unseen, unaffected by our words, untainted by our actions. I would say this is where blind faith to me was real and necessary.

Blind faith in reasoning, however, eventually wore down my reliance on the religion that I once knew. There was an entanglement of truth and perceptions that I was trying to untangle without really knowing what I was doing, but sensing that I was doing the right thing for me. Guilt from a betrayal of unity saddened me at times. It bore down heavily upon me while I came to terms with the fact that I was changing fundamentally from within. If I retreated in any way from how I felt, I would not have been true to myself. I was alone on this endeavor to be sure, but that is how it should be, really. Where else is strength gained more than from within?

A finely scrolled antique silver cross that I acquired in California stays with me so I don't forget. It is black with tarnish now, but to me, even more handsome. It symbolizes some very personal feelings I will never abandon; I respect it. I keep it with me as a reminder of what once was. I've been told that good men seldom deny their past; so I won't.

I suppose that I'm alright with this only because I truly do understand what is happening to me, which can only come about on my own—far away from the influences of tradition. I began to see that there were things meant to be obtained in the company of others, and there are also things meant to be gained—alone. I just felt it was right for me. I have always been a pathfinder in life; I saw this as no different.

I thought about the many ways life had shown me change as one of its conditions, which made me remember that when there is an end, a new beginning always follows. What new beginning awaits me? Will I ever know this everlasting presence that has always been there with me? I know there is something real ahead for me.

Through the years I lived with something guiding me and the knowledge that there is more than one can see out there. It is a force that bonds, heals, empowers, and can also humble us. We can never own it but it is there for us always. I have liberated myself and therefore have left room for what I am certain is there but have not yet entirely understood. I am humbled with hope that I will be united with this inner feeling of God. My strength comes from the confidence of being able to stand alone, especially when this ability is so far from what I have lived in the past.

And when asked if I pray, I say that my actions in life are my prayers. My prayers are movements—of grace, offering and contributions.

This, I will tell them, for now, is my religion.

THE PATH
TO CALIFORNIA

For a time I was far from steady—in mind, health, and in spirit. My thoughts led me in many directions as my reality set a much harder course for the immediate future. As much as it was not what I wanted, it was the only deliberate certainty in my life, and I had to deal with it. The complications that plagued me from the radical therapies I had been exposed to made it impossible to escape the past or move on. It seemed like I was caught in limbo. Whenever I would make any strides, I encountered another setback and was forced to be patient, yet again. It was wearing. Being physically compromised, emotionally frustrated, and spirituality exhausted further isolated me. I dug in and endured whatever came to me—and it came. I fought for my life through those years like I've never fought for anything else. I relied heavily on my nurses to have my back when I was at my weakest.

My body bore so much pain that it became tolerant to extremes. I began to realize that I could temper my reaction to it if I convinced myself that I could handle it. I was not one to reach for medication at the first sign of pain, but I knew that I had to break its cycle, eventually. The only difference would be that I would be the one to make the decision—not the pain. This way I stayed in control in an unpredictable environment.

Trickles of relief from the ongoing complications came to me in my dreams. I dreamed of ordinary things when I could and gloriously when I dared. And if I was fortunate enough, there were times when my dreams brought to me the dearest of my memories, those of my childhood, when life was no way near as serious. That was as good as it got.

I never stopped wanting a better life for myself; I never gave up hope that things would improve. But my hope was far from idle; I was willing to do something about it, even if it meant changing further from what had already changed so much in my life. I had so many more questions than answers and I wouldn't allow myself to rest until the opposite was true. It was the only way I would quiet the voices in my head that desperately longed for clarity, purpose, and a sense of spirituality.

The cancer was gone, the poisons had been put away, but I was far from out of the woods, because I hadn't gotten myself together, respectfully.

It was such a strong feeling for me—not being normal—that it caused me not to think of who I'd be leaving behind, should I follow my urges. It wasn't the only reason that I did what I did, but it stood out among them. After years of separation and a fair amount of self-analysis, the one thing I craved the most was to blend back into the mainstream of society as if nothing had happened. The lure of normality was very influential. I wanted others not to see the cancer that shadowed me. I thought that if I had tried to reconnect with my friends, I wasn't convinced this would happen. I didn't have that kind of confidence. I wasn't even sure they would want to be with me again. I set my sights on a distant horizon. I thought I could get away with this notion somewhere far from where I was, somewhere promising, fresh and new to me. Preferring warmth over the cold, I thought I might follow the sun while I was at it; so I faced myself westward, towards a genial coastline, and there it was—California.

I took along many truths of my experience that I held close while in my new environment. Personally, I had come a long way. Yet, I still needed the intimacy of relations. With all that I had been through and learned, there was something missing that I couldn't quite understand.

That something would prove to be more elusive than I could've ever imagined.

I fled aimlessly because of this sense of separation, hoping that distance would bring me closer. It seems contradictory—to go so far in order to be closer—but this feeling of being different from everyone who knew me distorted my sense of perception. I still lacked the confidence of realizing the worth of what I had lived through. I wasn't consciously aware that I was running from something or even chasing an illusion, but there was definitely a feeling of needing to escape, desperately coursing through my mind. I'm not proud of the fact that I gave in to such an impulse because this tends to wear down someone's confidence towards life. You can't run from something that is a part of you. You can't deny who you are or what you've been through. Until I fully appreciated this, it was exactly what I tried to do.

California proved to be all that I had hoped it would be. It took me far away from my past. I flourished. I attended classes in Los Angeles and San Luis Obispo. With extended family scattered across the state, I was able to see my young cousins' mature right before my eyes into commendable women. I had been to them the big brother they never had. It was a satisfying feeling. I had more than my share of friends and relationships to partially numb myself from my hospital memories. In some ways this was healing. I guess I really did need this in a way to sort of balance the extremes of my life. In this manner California provided that balance.

There were things that going to California could not offer me, even though it smiled on me and welcomed this stranger, things that can only come from within. I sensed that my stay had served its purpose when thoughts of these inner deficits of mine outweighed the benefits of being away. When this happened, I knew then that it was time to go home. Besides, I was more than ready to see my family again. I left them behind in the wake of my recovery, hoping they would understand my selfishness. They did because they loved me.

There was a certain obligation I felt to involve them in the life I was trying to piece together. But more than anything else—I missed them.

Driving cross country gave me plenty of time to think. One thought dominated all others. *Why was I still alone?* I kept asking myself. It was a question that wouldn't pass as systematically as the different states I drove through on my way home. It stayed with me for thousands of miles. It drowned out the radio no matter how loud I turned it. I realized that I was leaving everyone behind who entered into my life. After all these years, I still longed for true camaraderie. I needed someone to get it, whatever I was feeling inside that brought me closer to a kind of life that appreciated exalted sentiments, a life that demanded more from each one of us. At this point, I found myself grasping at the higher-self that I had discovered during my earlier struggles. No amount of everyday living could ever sustain this standard of life. I was beginning to expect this of myself and nothing else would be good enough. Whatever it was back then that showed me what was possible needed to be nurtured. It was alive in me and wanting. I began to notice the great distance between what it represented and what I was encountering around me.

There was an unseen threshold between me and most everyone else who entered into my life. It was a line not so easily crossed. I had changed by seeing what I couldn't see before my illness. It was a feeling that kept me within an arm's reach away from anyone.

So there it was, right in front of me. I was still isolated, even in the midst of so many. There was no denying the fact that I saw the world through different eyes. But it was the world that I desired to be close to. I could not go back to this sense of belonging unless I brought with me what I had become. The conflict of wanting both lives had to be settled. If ever I would find a way home, I would have to do it taking with me who and what I was—completely, proudly, and unconditionally. All this time I had been concerned about how I would be perceived. I was stuck in this rut. My identity is what mattered most. I was affected because I had a fixed idea of myself. I was not living with truth but a truth that had already passed. I was trying to be someone that I wasn't anymore. My mind wasn't living in the moment. I then realized that I had to lose this notion of my "self", my identity—if you will, in order to be unaffected by vanity, loss, and change. *Was this possible?* I wondered. *How would I go about this?*

The notes I had carried with me to and from California became the only connection to my past. I never let them leave my side, no matter where life took me. I felt a need to keep them. Maybe, in a way, what I had written was better pieces of myself that I had discovered. Maybe in those notes was who I really was beyond the petty layers of our ego; and that is why I held on so tightly to them, even though I had turned away from where I'd been.

I wasn't ready to read them—until I returned from California. There was enough distance in my mind from that time that I could now—comfortably—look back. After I pored through the scribbled notes, I started to understand why they meant so much to me. They had captured what my mind—out of self-preservation—could not hold onto. Many things that I had forgotten had resurfaced through this trail of words. The memories rushed to me and I began to connect the dots. It was coming back to me.

During this time, I gained a new respect for the human spirit. It was as if I was reading about someone else—at another time and place. I was taken aback by my resourcefulness and resilience. There was talk of struggle that was heartfelt, raw emotions that inspired as well as paralyzed the senses. I had thoughts that were provoking, and evocative dreams that lent me passage from the hardest times. I knew now why these notes had to be saved, because they were more than me. They weren't mine anymore than the mystery or the higher laws in life were exclusive to me. They belonged to the world. The human spirit—I find—transcends individuality.

So much can be lost in time; it heals in this way. But in that healing we can let go of some very important lessons. I wasn't about to let this happen. I had lived deliberately then and I wanted what was gained through that. I didn't have the right to forget some things. I wouldn't have been responsible to others had this happened. I was drawn by this force—this higher law; it exists beyond my ego. Sometimes it calls on you to be self-sacrificing. I could hear that call much louder than before.

I took on that challenge, a challenge by life to capture those fleeting truths that I had lived. I was ready for it then. It made sense to me now, much more than before.

I sorted through my notes for some semblance of order as I scattered the papers across the kitchen table. I wasn't sure where to start. I never knew it would be such a long road from that moment, but it turned out to be.

I looked at those thoughts on paper as I would so many pieces to a puzzle, each piece seemingly insignificant, yet essential to seeing the whole picture.

I was missing some of those pieces that would bring everything together. I was soon to find out they were the most important pieces of all, and I would've been lost without them. A chance encounter would present them to me; a chance encounter with Charlene.

CHARLENE

It was autumn of '93; I returned home in time to see the foliage flaunt its most striking pose. The atmosphere was crisp with hints of winter to come. The sun's warmth was distant except for when it was at its highest in the sky and the clouds weren't in its way. Only then was there a brief reminder of summers past, and for me, California's lenient seasons. Change was near.

Not everyone can say in this temporal life that they've walked with a giant; even fewer can say that they've changed because of this. Some of us may only get one chance to chase something passionately before life's attracting spell wears off and all that we are left with is regret. As the years went on I began to think that with all that I had been through, this promise of passion and beauty wasn't meant for me, that somehow it might elude me. That was, until I met her.

During one of my first breaks from writing I did something very much out of the ordinary. I turned on the television for some company. Walking back to the kitchen table which doubled as my desk, was the first time I heard her voice; I sensed the unusual silence of her audience. It was *her* audience; anyone could see this.

There was something serious happening and I had just walked in on it—if you will.

After she spoke, I stopped what I was doing and quickly knelt in front of the television to get a better view, anticipating more. She definitely had caught my interest. I could see right away how there was something special about this woman, something that set her apart from the others sitting next to Charlene. It wasn't about beauty as much as it was about stoicism, she was forthright and unwavering. Just listening to her speak was enough for me to conclude this. This woman, this stranger to me, was able to bring forth a sense of living truth that had been missing in my life after my recovery from cancer.

Charlene's venturesome eyes sparkled like two confident diamonds. My heart pounded with excitement and anticipation that I might have found someone so close to the way that I felt inside. My spirit came alive with hope that I had come across what I thought I might never find in my lifetime.

All this was racing through my mind as she spoke deliberately of her breast cancer with the conviction of a warrior. Her voice was steady and sure of its words as they delivered their message to the attentive crowd. I could see many traits of myself in her. Charlene looked at this much the way that I did. She was fighting in a war I had twice weathered against a familiar adversary.

Charlene explained how she dealt with having breast cancer and then spoke of how, at the age of twenty-seven she was taking her relapse in stride. She told those who would listen that cancer was with her but didn't have her; she was still in control of her life.

Every word hit home. I could see that we were nearly the same age, but more importantly, her attitude reflected mine so well. I also noticed—as one who's been told many times the same—the devil in her eyes; they were wildly untamed and captivatingly daring, revealing an edge of defiant undertones, harboring just a tinge of glistening mischief behind them. If I was a gambler I'd bet she wanted it that way. How well we know what we are familiar with.

Charlene was letting the world into her spirit; her eyes were wide open—like windows without shades. She was inviting us to be a part of her plight by this candid disclosure. It was her way of making us aware how deeply women were suffering from this terrible disease, and that something needed to be done about it soon. Hers was an urgent theme.

I knelt in front of the screen, wanting to hear more. I couldn't get enough. I saw something in her that reminded me of when I too traveled along that road of the unknown. I missed that heightened sense of awareness that I had left somewhere in the past, an awareness and appreciation for life that only a brush with death can arouse. To have it so near that your heart beats out of your chest. To be erect in spirit and defy fear in the face of a threat having such finality as it breathes its cold breath against your will and bones, summons all of your vitality to the forefront of your existence. The hairs on your body raise on end and every god given sense bestowed on you is flushed with attention to the moment, during which there is no doubt that you are living fully awake. At one time I knew how that felt, to be that aware of the intensity where life and death merge—or more—collide. Watching this unfold made me remember how real life can be.

After the show I was left with an urge to contact Charlene. I wanted so much to let her know I heard what she said; I wanted to show her that she wasn't alone. You may come across a thousand pretty faces and even more inviting smiles, but every now and then there is one who brings the sun, the beauty of a flower captured in the crest of bloom, or even the mystery of eternity caught deep within the eyes. The ones who are truly blessed are those who notice, for that makes all the difference in the world.

I wanted to know Charlene personally. Something told me that she was inhaling the very essence of life; she was living in the moment where an undeniable truth can only be found. Living this way awakens a hunger for life that is not so easily satisfied in our culture. Seeing her determination to not give in fully inspired me. This came at a time when I was finally ready to reach out, unlike the many years I had kept to myself, where I had found there to be no lasting strength.

It wasn't very long before I drew up enough courage to find her. I made up my mind to do what I have wanted to do for many years, and that was to step back into life's rude den. But this time, I would have a seasoned will, and it would be for all-together different reasons. I wanted fear, guilt, doubt and self-preservation to be replaced with purpose, compassion and selflessness. I had changed, and part of that change was to understand the need to interact in a way which comforts and eases others beside myself.

I wasn't willing to risk losing a chance to bond with someone I had been searching for, someone who might need me in this very way, a way in which others could not reach me, no matter how hard they tried or how much I hoped they could. In order to do this I would need to take that first step.

The only thing I could remember that might help me find Charlene was hearing her sister Julie refer to her profession in the radiology department at a hospital in Philadelphia. It wasn't much to go on, but it was all that I had. I dialed information only to find out there were several hospitals in the vicinity. The operator held while I thought about it. Finally I asked her to give me the first two. I then picked one and proceeded to phone the radiology department. A woman answered. I asked for Julie. "Which one, there are two?" She replied. *I couldn't believe it.* "The one with a sister named Charlene." I said. That did it. She told me to hold on. The next voice I heard was Julie's—the right one. I explained to her that I had just seen Charlene on television and I wanted to send her a card to wish her well and somehow let her know that she touched me. "I had been through something similar." I told Julie.

Well, I will tell you, I got way more than I bargained for. Julie invited me to call her sister personally. Charlene was staying at her house while undergoing treatments. I felt privileged and eagerly anticipated the conversation, thinking about what might be said to break the ice. I even wondered whether she would care to get involved with a stranger, knowing what she was going through. Fighting for someone's life is a very personal thing and I completely understood if she wasn't interested. I remember wanting very much to be alone most of the time when I was ill. But she seemed different. Regardless, I was going to try. I wanted to reach out—I needed to reach out.

That same night, I called Charlene; she answered. I guess it was a bit awkward, but she made me feel comfortable right away. That was part of her beautiful personality. We talked for nearly three hours. I learned enough about her to want very much to pursue a friendship. I would like to think the feeling was mutual, but I was never the pushy type so I waited for her to decide what might come of this. As we said our goodbyes, she asked if I would call her again. Of course I told her that I would.

For almost a year we kept this going strong, as I would always let her set the pace and tone of the conversation. Whenever she wasn't up to it—that was all right too. It was all about Charlene to me. I let her be herself and say anything she wanted to, and trust me she did, holding nothing back. We laughed hard at times, often about the silliest things, but mostly, we would bust on the current events of the day, whatever we could improvise with, so long as I was taking her away for a while. We never took much seriously.

If this meant that I ended up in Charlene's humor-laced crosshairs, so be it. She could take it as well, which made it even more challenging because I also enjoyed dishing it out. We would go round and round, often getting so out of hand that we weren't sure anymore where the boundaries were or even who had crossed them, but neither one of us cared. I think that she got a kick out of me, and I really liked her. Not in the way one might think; come to think of it, you know, I never really thought about Charlene in a girlfriend way, that wasn't something that I considered. Our phone calls never took on that kind of atmosphere, but we did innocently play with innuendo from time to time.

Charlene was like a breath of fresh air. Much of her authenticity came natural to her, because she was already living the higher laws. A clear indication of this was her ability to welcome into her world an outsider, such as myself.

As time went by, I couldn't wait to call her. I couldn't wait to hear her say, "Hey you..." in that low inviting tone of hers. This may not seem like a big deal, but I have found that little things like that can be the sweetest part of living. We all hunger for such subtle gestures of intimacy. They can make us feel so good inside, so welcome.

Charlene's voice was distinct. I had never heard a woman speak so softly yet command such attention. She definitely had that "it" factor. She had presence, even on the phone.

Her laugh provoked me into finding any reason to cause her to. It was as evocative and unusual as she was. I could never mistake Charlene for another. Her voice was her signature. Perhaps I'm a bit biased; it was what bonded us from the start.

Charlene would never ask who it was when I phoned; she recognized me right away, and she had many friends. If she received another call while we were talking, which wasn't uncommon, she wouldn't take it until we had hung up. What is that worth to someone? To me it spoke volumes about her attention and commitment to the moment. And whenever the idea struck her, I would be lucky enough to hear that crazy noise her mini dachshund Sophie made when she was rubbed between the ears. I couldn't help but crackup.

Sophie meant the world to her. I often thought about what would happen to her little companion should something terrible come to pass. I didn't want to think about it, but sometimes your mind wanders down the road of the future like a leash-less puppy, especially when you care so much.

Charlene possessed so many unique qualities worthy of mention. One of them was her ability to remember the details of our conversation. If I wasn't on the ball she would call me on it and, you know, she was always right. She was such a good listener who knew how to hold your attention. Charlene was dynamic. She could still be her polite self while gracefully delivering sarcastic blows that would rival a prize fighter.

Her words that followed were like a cold sirloin slapped on your ego. Boy, could she humble a guy with her wit. I loved that about her.

How rare is it to have so many layers and each be approachable, especially when one's life is so distracted on such a serious level?

We bonded within a short span of time, but I don't feel that time is in play when it comes to this kind of closeness. In fact time tends to stand still when two find a place to run free and rejoice under the great blanket of trust and friendship, where the only breach of that haven would be if one of us were to blink. It is as if you were incredibly happy and then suddenly you became aware of this happiness, where then it abruptly leaves you. This feeling was usually a phone hang-up away; a sobering reality that often brought me back to the truth of the situation and its cold hard facts.

Many nights after hanging up with her I would just sit there staring into nowhere, thinking about what she was feeling, what she must be going through, almost at times putting myself in her situation. It was becoming personal. So many nights I thought about calling her back because I had wanted to say this or that about what I thought might be running through her mind. I never did. I was afraid that I might have opened a Pandora's Box, a movement that would have brought me so much closer to the flames. I lost those moments, those possibilities, and I have to live with that. I have to live with the fact that I hesitated. I could've been stronger.

On the other hand, I also understood from the very beginning that I was in Charlene's theater. I held to that conviction with a deep respect for her privacy. There was so much I could have said that I let go, never to be heard by her. I trusted that she knew where I had been, and if there was something she thought about asking me, she would have. Sometimes I felt a staunch obligation to measure the moment for appropriateness.

To know and have confidence in others means that there must be an ability to restrain, to have patience, even when it's your natural inclination to advise or lead. When I met Charlene I had a raw knowledge of myself and what I had lived through, but so much was still missing. I wasn't aware that she was a big part of what was missing. So little did I know! Besides, the things I could've showed her, had she inquired, Charlene was already living, more intensely than I might ever have. I think I was beginning to see that this was much more than my relationship with her; there was something significant happening here. Charlene was able to escape the stigma surrounding her life and relation with family and her close friends by reaching out to a stranger who wasn't there in the trenches, as they were and had been since the beginning. This opportunity came directly to her, while I searched far and wide for mine. That gave me a little insight into why I may have left all who knew me and headed for California. I understood her in this way.

Charlene was getting more from me than I had ever thought I could give her and I was learning more about myself in the process. She was relating to the world through me, as if she had never fallen ill. Knowing me was giving her a chance to live out that possibility. By not bringing her health into our conversations, we made sure of this. My voice—a stranger's voice—opened the door to another life, a life that might have been if things were different for her.

My sleep was often restless during our friendship, but that didn't bother me. I was beginning to realize how close I was getting to Charlene, and I understood what this meant. It meant that eventually I would have to deal with our meeting in person. Charlene often dropped subtle hints as to when I would come to see her. She would say that things might change with her condition, but never pressed the issue. I think she may have thought my reluctance to commit was due to the fact that we lived far from each other, but the distance in miles wasn't the problem. It was, I'm ashamed to say, emotional distance on my part. Something stopped me from completely committing to Charlene. I felt somewhat safe the way things were. I guess this was one of the many reasons why she was a giant, and I a simple human. The fearlessness that once defined me while I was fighting for my life during my time in isolation waned at the hand of the many distractions in society. I lost sight of that bold attitude that forged ahead without pause.

This contrast of strength and fear that I held within my mind simmered for years. I hadn't understood why there was this inner conflict or why I could be so courageous back then and hesitant later. Was something lost or just latent in me? Maybe this is why I searched for someone like Charlene. Maybe all along I was thirsting for purpose in life. When there is purpose—meaningful purpose, fear flees the scene. At one time I knew this feeling very well and I think that I have been chasing it ever since. Life reveals reason in many basic forms, it can be found anywhere at any time. But purpose is a higher law, and much more driven are we when we have it; it's the one thing that compels the spirit to reach for new heights.

I needed Charlene more than I had realized. I was drawn to her for reasons that at the time I wasn't even aware of. I still had yet to come into my own; maybe I foresaw what lay ahead for her and it was simply too much for me to handle. I do know that my family was often concerned that I might get hurt in some way should something happen to Charlene. They were only looking out for me, but I think their cautiousness infected me.

I stalled for as long as I could before Charlene made the decision for me. In the end, it was her sincerity that gave me the guts to go to Philadelphia and meet with her. One particular conversation is what made the difference. Charlene was being her normal self, delivering a dash of wit speckled over some of her lighthearted observations. I agreed with her. Then she was silent, just long enough to get my full attention. When she was sure she had mine, Charlene spoke; "You know, if you are thinking of seeing me David, I wouldn't wait any longer."

That's all that it took for me. No other words said in any other way could have come as close to my heart with such deep penetration. We both could have spent the next year figuring out what time would have been convenient, or time might have snuck up on us and stole any chance we might've had to see each other before I was ready. Charlene swiftly broke this impasse by knowing exactly what to say and how to say it.

We were both anxious to see one another once I committed to a date. She would tell me how she couldn't believe we were finally going to meet each other, and how she could hardly wait. I thought about our meeting—a lot.

I knew what Charlene looked like, but she had never seen me. She would say that it was unfair to her. Not that it really mattered, but we all know how that goes. I still thought about what Charlene would think of me physically. I was so thin from the effects of the therapies on my system. Now and then vanity crept into my consciousness. This would happen mostly when it came to the other gender. To this I say that nobody's perfect, I guess.

I boarded a train in Providence bound for Philadelphia. I was on my way. I arrived at the station in Philly some hours later, after a long jostling ride. My anticipation overshadowed any inconvenience I might have had. Once I stepped off the train, the only thing that really mattered was seeing her. The first impression Charlene gave me was a warm welcoming smile. I was later told that she prayed I wasn't too unbearably hideous. I was pleased to find out that she exhaled with relief after we had actually met. I on the other hand, knew just what I was getting, and was not at all disappointed. In fact, Charlene impressed me even more, showing up on a motorcycle that her father had recently bought for her. She had always wanted one, and was finally able to live out one of her dreams. It was quite a sight to see as she walked toward me, dressed in black leather motorcycle chaps over faded jeans, with black leather riding boots. A dressy white shirt polished off the outfit, and she was all it. I managed to remain outwardly composed, but inside I shook like a silly fan wanting an autograph.

I was there with her after more than a year of phone calls; we had finally met in person. No longer did I have the barrier of distance to protect me in some way. I was committed to this experience whether I liked it or not.

I followed her home in a taxi while she led the way on her motor-cycle, taking us to a row of brick buildings with cobblestone roads within the great city of Philadelphia—Center City, to be exact. The weekend was ahead of us, and I wondered where this opportunity would take us, and also what it would present us. At first, my thoughts were simple. I thought about seeing her favorite playmate, Sophie—wondering if she would take to me.

Charlene's apartment was warm, and full of character. It had a steep loft, which was her bedroom. I remember looking up there and wishing I had the privacy of a loft when I needed it, somewhere to escape, just to get away. The whole time I was there, I never saw that room, nor did I give it a thought thereafter. The stairs to her retreat were abrupt, narrow and mysterious.

I figured that many of her vintage personal belongings that she had mentioned during our conversations adorned that loft, and that maybe someday I might see them. But this was also Charlene's private sanctuary. I respected that.

I had my hands full anyway with Sophie; she took to me right away. She was getting to know me and wanted my undivided attention. I guess she accepted me as Charlene's friend. There were play toys scattered about that Charlene would have me tug from Sophie to hear those crazy sounds she made to me over the phone. That little dog was a hoot. I could easily see how Charlene could get so attached to her. Charlene watched and laughed as her vicious attack dog had her way with me until we—Sophie and I—decided on a truce. To seal the deal, Sophie leaped in my arms and proceeded to coat my face with doggie saliva.

I was just beginning to settle down in this new environment, so far away from my home and everything that I was familiar with. I could tell that Charlene was not one to remain idle for very long, so we set off down the narrow side streets of Center City, passing interesting shops and eateries along the way. We were both antique junkies. We came upon a special vintage store of hers which Charlene proudly declared her favorite. She then eagerly grasped my hand and quickly led me in. It was a refreshingly genuine experience for me to see this woman so excited to just be alive, to be so enthralled with the simple things in life. It made her that much more beautiful to me.

The nearing sun of late spring warmed the cobblestones, causing shimmering heat to rise from the gently, toasted stones. Brilliant flashes of light danced off the hoods of cars and against shop windows, poking through the secret alleyways which led to legitimate speak-easies that would spring alive well into the night. They overflowed with patrons who had been waiting all week long to mix and mingle with old friends and new acquaintances. There were many people around us on this Saturday. The atmosphere was festive. I thought this a bit unusual for just any old weekend, but didn't bother to mention it to her. After all, I was in a big city, much bigger than Providence, and wasn't sure what was normal here.

Charlene *knew* why the streets were crowded, but she wasn't about to tell me, not yet anyway. We had just stepped out of a chocolate and candy store when she noticed the time slipping by us. She took hold of the moment right away, as she hurried us toward the water's edge, just ahead. It was so becoming to see her turn back to me, so full of the moment, to press my pace.

The closer we got to the water, the more people I saw. I could hear, off in the distance, a voice singing. The words were still unclear to me, yet very soothing. As we neared the commotion a monumental amphitheater appeared, poised proudly with the bay as its background. Charlene looked at me and smiled. I was surprised and delighted. I had never been to a concert like this.

She asked if I recognized the performer.

"No, who is she?" I replied.

"Sarah McLachlan," she answered. I wasn't familiar with her then, but watched her climb to stardom in the years that followed my visit with Charlene. I listened to Sarah's beautiful voice while we looked around for Charlene's friends who were to meet us there. They saved seats for us. I wasn't easily distracted from Charlene, but I was gripped by Sarah's angelic voice. To me, it captured the moment of my visit, perfectly. I felt so aligned with her mood and I could see from others around me that I wasn't alone. We were all entranced. The next couple of hours were enriching. I enjoyed every minute of it.

After we had been there for some time, Charlene began to feel tired, so we said our goodbyes and headed back home. I offered to get a taxi, but she was determined to return the same way she came—on foot. I loved that in her; it revealed so much about her spirit. By the time we arrived at her apartment, Charlene desperately needed some rest. She excused herself and then slowly made her way up the loft. Sophie and I watched her disappear up the shadowy stairs of her retreat, both missing her already.

The late afternoon sun was, by now, straight across from the living room windows. Its warmth squeezed between and through the pulled back curtains, momentarily hypnotizing the both of us. I fell back into the couch as my eyelids struggled to stay open. Sophie climbed on my chest and nestled herself in a comfortable position. It took a couple of passes before she was actually satisfied.

The room stilled.

A little while later, Sophie hopped off me in excitement as she heard scuffling upstairs. That meant her mistress had awakened. She could hardly contain herself as she ran to the stairs in an effort to hasten the reunion. I waited patiently, but was just as eager to be in Charlene's company again. I could see, as she carefully descended down the stairs, that her rest had been refreshing. She then sat next to me, smiling, congenially. I stood up a moment later. She watched me fidget emotionally as she sat there. I paced the floor knowing, sensing almost intuitively, that there was something on her mind. I peeked her way and felt the heaviness of her stare, as her eyes fixed on mine. Charlene was an engaging woman. Her eyes could draw you to her. I could not turn away from them. Then the words that broke an unspoken pact between us were delivered, with a child's sincerity and a woman's composure. Charlene spoke to me as if something was approaching and time made all the difference. Up until now, neither one of us had ever talked in any profound way about what we had been through. Both of us had managed to keep our conversations lighthearted and upbeat, skillfully maneuvering around trigger themes of dialogue. In the past, brief moments of concern had somehow wandered into our discussions, but we chased them away as fast as we could. This time would be no slipup. I could see that Charlene's mood was a pensive one.

"David…I know if anyone can understand what I'm feeling, it's you, she said. I can't imagine what it was like for you to go through this when you were so young. At least I'm a little older; I've had my teenage years to experience. Tell me…how did you get through this?"

She caught me off guard. I hesitated, reaching down to pet Sophie, stalling for a moment of recollection. Then I blurted out, "I looked at it like I did a challenge in sports, as something to be beaten."

I really didn't want to say what I did, but I also did not want to be coy. *I didn't come here to talk about me*, I thought to myself. And more than anything, I didn't want to distract her from this moment. It was Charlene's moment. I had secretly waited for so long to have this kind of dialogue with her; I wasn't about to influence its natural movement. I wanted Charlene to talk to me about what she was living through—what was going through her thoughts as she fought for her life. The truth was I could see that my situation, although it happened at a much earlier time in my life, was not as unforgiving as Charlene's predicament. So I resisted the idea of talking about my chance outcome. I didn't want to differentiate us in anyway. There was no need to.

I hoped that she wouldn't ask me to elaborate. But then, maybe this would somehow comfort her if I said the right thing. I did know that if pressed, I would never deny Charlene a candid answer. It didn't take much to understand why I was torn. All one had to do was see her from where I stood, as her immaculate, delicate, white, dress shirt opened just enough to reveal a bandage where her breast had recently been removed. There was no escaping the fact that I was witnessing a woman in the fight of her life. This left me almost verbally paralyzed, because it was difficult for me to see her so vulnerable. I had been raised to think of women as those to be protected. There was something so wrong about this. It was so unnatural to accept that Charlene would have to endure this suffering and still could die in the end.

Charlene held her stare, attempting to provoke a better response from me, as if to say, 'That's not fair; you and I know there's more.'

I shrugged my shoulders, as if to gesture that it was no big deal. I was humbled in her presence from the beginning. The last thing I wanted to do was tell how I had made it through, knowing full well that her chances were looking very slim. To see her tender frame before me, compared to when I first saw her on television more than a year ago, affected me. The reality of this human being that stood in front of me made me choose my words carefully. I felt as if I was fortunate to have survived. This made me no different than Charlene. I was no different than her. We are all a hair's breadth away from the same fate. The only distance we create is in our minds. Life is no less vital coming to these terms. If anything, it becomes much more vital, and makes you acutely aware of time.

I worried that in some way I was letting her down. But what was I supposed to say? What would have been the right words that might have made everything better for her? How do you choose your words in such a forum of spontaneity? Sometimes, to say nothing is to say everything.

By now Sophie was in her arms, and Charlene had all but abandoned her inquiry. There was silence again, though not the same silence that we had known before. I could tell that it was only a prelude to more, so I remained reluctantly ready, not knowing exactly what to expect. Charlene then gently released Sophie to the floor. She got up and stood next to the window, leaning her head and shoulders against the frame while peering toward the setting sun, though I could tell, mostly into her thoughts. The only sound was that of Sophie's tiny paws that pitter pattered across the hardwoods as she trailed Charlene to the window. Sophie's head tilted upward—trying to see her mistress, almost sensing the deep feeling in the room.

Still looking away through the glass, Charlene spoke softly of how there were many days and nights that she wrestled with the idea of death. She acknowledged that even though so many of her friends and family were with her, fully supporting her, so near to her that she could touch them, she knew that they could only come so far into the place where she was. She wondered how they could be so close and yet so distant, how life is peculiar this way. I saw a moment of melancholy come across her. It seemed as if she realized in some way, through this all, that she was alone.

"But I don't at all feel lonely." Charlene turned to me and declared, catching me reflecting on similar feelings. Her words were healing me from within. Thoughts I had shoved way back in the farthest corners of my mind were of this nature, and she had brought them to the present so easily. Charlene truly understood. She spoke to me from the center of her heart, and in doing so, pierced mine. I was drawn to her thoughts, to these sentiments, to her very attitude. She continued, trying to explain this stillness that comes forth in your mind, when truth slows to a lone cloud's pace in a cerulean sky and fear retreats into the abyss.

I showed little expression, nor did I say a word, but she could tell that I knew just what she meant. Her words resonated. My God, how I could relate to this. I was so relieved. From then on I knew that Charlene had found that familiar place that I had retreated to in my time of need. It was where I had found an enormous peace in the face of danger. I could never describe it, but remembered it very well and how calming it was to my spirit. I could see now that it was the same way with her, just by what she was saying and—more importantly—by the way she had said it.

Charlene turned to me gently, almost forgivingly, and told how there was a dark, grave concern in the eyes of those near to her heart. She could see this in them, even though they tried to hide their concern. Still gazing outward, she went on:

"But I wonder David, I wonder if they're aware of the brilliant activity that is in my imagination—if they realize how I feel that I have somehow lived before? I wonder if they know that for some reason I'm not sad. I believe that I will live again. I wonder if somehow they will remember me beyond my last days, and maybe think of me the way that I could have been?

They are right there with me, watching what I'm watching—but they do not see what I see. You know…in my mind I've glimpsed the eternal. There's something more out there. It might be waiting for me. It waits for all of us. That calms me David. When I look back to see if there are regrets—I have none. I'm giving all that I can give and really couldn't ask anymore of myself. If I don't make it, it's OK. I'm alright with that now."

I wanted to hold her right then, but that was not the time. She was in the middle of a brave moment. She owned it. That moment deserved respect. I held back for a time and then firmly exclaimed, "No."

Charlene looked at me for a moment, and then looked away, gently dismissing my reaction.

Without a single word spoken, I was put in my place. These were her thoughts; I was just there to witness.

She looked down at her pride and joy. "I don't know what you'll do without me, Sophie; I worry about you so much. I would miss you terribly."

As unannounced as it came, the moment was gone.

Charlene asked if I was hungry. Her confident smirk returned as she began to describe this fun little crab shack nestled by the Chesapeake Bay. Her eyes gleamed with excitement. I was starved and loved crabs too, so I nodded in agreement.

By now it was dusk and the streets were no longer lighted by the sun, but by old-fashioned lamp posts. The warm glow of neon was visible in the windows of the local bar and grills'. A tarot card reader and some shops remained opened for the evening crowd to wander in—I would say, more for idle entertainment than anything else. The store owners provided quaint geniality as they bantered with passersby.

I had never had so much fun at a restaurant in my life as I did that night. It was literally a feeding frenzy. Everyone there was in on it. We acted like kids. It was a war zone of spent shells piled high in front of her and me. They were all over the floor as well. I'm pretty sure that was the idea, but 'til this day I couldn't say for certain whether we broke some rules of etiquette or not. All that I know is we weren't the only ones making a complete mess.

We were well into the evening, and after washing our hands with about a dozen or so of those silly wipes, we finally managed to get rid of the smell. But it was well worth it.

Charlene wanted to visit some friends who were having a get together close by, so off we went. It was there that I met some pretty impressive people, who called Charlene their friend. She introduced me as a writer, but I quickly added that I was nothing of the sort. She overruled my modesty, and reaffirmed that I was a writer. Charlene knew enough to save me from my own insecurity and I wasn't going to dispute that. We relaxed for the rest of the night.

I grabbed a taxi to get us home because I knew how tired Charlene was, even though she would have never admitted it. I told her that

I was pretty beat, and felt like getting a ride instead of walking. She called me a lightweight, but I think she knew that I was always thinking about her. That was classic Charlene at her best.

On the way home, she asked me if I would want to go sailing on Sunday with her parents, who had invited us. I had never sailed before; I've been on boats many times, but never really sailed. "Of course I'll go," I told her.

The morning brought an abundance of clouds and plenty of promising winds to fill our prospective sails. I was hoping that the day would be as memorable as the one before. I would be leaving the next morning.

Charlene rode me on her motorcycle all the way there, a good twenty-five minute ride. Her mom and dad were waiting for us on the boat, all ready to set sail by the time we had arrived. It was the first time I had seen her parents. Charlene's father impressed me with his stature. He was a big man with a sturdy build. Right away I could see that this man was to be admired by other men, for his presence.

Once on the boat, it took close to forty-five minutes to actually reach the mouth of the Chesapeake, as we slowly navigated the heavily horsefly-infested marshes. I made the mistake of positioning myself in the bow during this dreadful passageway while everyone else wisely retreated to the lower deck. I spent that whole time frantically swatting enormous flies. There had to be literally hundreds swarming around me at any given time. I'm sure that I looked like a complete lunatic, but the worst of it came when one of my senseless swats sent my expensive sunglasses into the murky water. My heart sank in sync with my glasses, as I watched them quickly disappear. Fortunately, as we neared the mouth of the bay, the horseflies vanished.

The open water was amazing. I sat there in the bow, hovering overhead as the hull sliced into the choppy currents beneath me. I felt so free. Once in a while I glanced back to Charlene and she would smile in return, letting me know everything was all right. I thought I might give her and her parents some time alone and, to be honest, I was really enjoying the view from where I was.

The remainder of the day was thought-filled. It was quiet and the mood was a pensive one. The sun finally retreated behind the distant array of fish-scale clouds, which are often a prelude to rain. We all did our own thinking in silence; none of us were in the moment for very long. There might have been a brief wink or two between us, but it was obvious there was so much more going on there than an afternoon of sailing. I would see Charlene at times embrace her mom and dad and then look off into the sea. Her father struck me as a simple and silent man. I could see that he was the rock in the family; Charlene leaned on him from time to time. It wasn't hard to see where his vulnerability was. I once called Charlene Charlie. Her voice softened. "That's what my dad sometimes calls me," she said. He meant so much to her. I didn't say it again.

Charlene's mom was like my own mother. She had a gentle strength that one could notice when she spoke. She was an insightful person. Josephine was more Charlene's friend than anything else; they often related to each other like sisters. I had heard her voice now and then when I talked to Charlene on the phone. She would interject her thoughts into our conversations, and they were welcome. When Charlene was too hard on me, Jo would tell her to leave me alone. It was fun. Charlene always spoke fondly of her mother. She loved her so.

There was no doubt that, on that boat, that day, the three of them were as close as family can be. I felt privileged to see this. All in all, it was a memorable, surreal day. We said our goodbyes and journeyed home.

The last night I was with Charlene we talked a bit more about women, breast cancer, and her thoughts about the unnatural combination. She told me the one thing she wanted was to offer impoverished women a chance to maintain their beauty and dignity while going through treatments. Charlene wanted these women to be able to have wigs as they lost their hair and makeup to cover their pallid complexions caused by the unflattering effects of radiation and chemotherapy. This was very important to Charlene because she realized how a woman's femininity can be compromised in such a way. She also reasoned that to feel good about oneself in this way would reflect on one's attitude within as well. Once that was not an issue, then a woman could focus on the fighting for life part.

Charlene hoped that one day there would be a thriving fund in her name that would somehow cater to this seemingly incidental need of women enduring breast cancer.

Charlene treated me to a home-cooked meal that night, as she told me how fond she was of the culinary arts. It was refreshing to have someone else prepare my meal for once. All I had to do was enjoy it. I wasn't accustomed to this, but could see myself easily getting used to it.

After dinner, we sat in the living room and talked more about what mattered to her. Knowing that I would be leaving the next morning, Charlene was eager to talk more about what she wanted to say in this book. I told her she had the freedom to say whatever she felt. I was so proud to offer her this.

What struck me the most was her willingness to see past her death. That took strength and maturity. Charlene was eager to leave something behind. I think she understood even then that she held a gift which was meant to be opened by the world, not just her friends and family. There was something special and attractive about her that was never meant to be bound by chance or circumstance. I'm sure that if her fate had been different, Charlene would have lived mightily, and would have affected many people, as she did me and those around her. Her mind was already vast and expansive, encountering life from moment to moment. Within her spirit all the secrets of immortality were held, though this immortality was not borne of vanity. It was a longing for the one thing death was denying her, a relationship with the world. Charlene wasn't quite sure what was to come, but she did know that it couldn't smother her spirit.

Once we trod on our unspoken pact, the subject came to us quite easily. Our relationship had changed. We had moved closer through handling a delicate matter so well. There was respect.

We both thought aloud about the days ahead. Charlene's doctors were preparing her for some very intense treatments in the near future, and her health might suddenly take a turn for the worse.

I never saw fear in Charlene's eyes—even then. They were fixed in the moment, with an exceptional reflection of life within them. No one would ever believe she had been through so much. If I gazed long enough directly into her eyes, I'm sure that I would've seen forever. They remained serene through it all, like two fathomless pools of infinite poise, undaunted by and impervious to any omen cast upon Charlene.

She had a knack for keeping things in perspective. Here was a woman in her twenties who had not opened the precious gift of motherhood or promised herself in a way that would bond her with one man for life. Instead she was fighting desperately for her own life. Yet, you could never sense this deprivation, because Charlene lived with you in the here and now; she never wasted a moment in the past.

On the morning I was to leave, Charlene thanked me for coming and asked if it was worth the effort. I just smiled; she smiled back. On the way home I realized that I was a different person than before I visited her. I no longer thought of where I had been raised my whole life as my 'home'. Home took on a new meaning for me. I felt like I could be anywhere and still be at *home*; that is, if purpose followed me. This is the affect Charlene had on me; this is how she made me feel. She made me feel like my life was vast, boundless and meaningful. As long as there were people like Charlene in the world, I would be all right—no matter where I was. She was the best reflection of truth that I had found so far.

It was the beginning of a new era for me; one that would dramatically alter the manner in which I relate in the world. Charlene was changing me in ways that no amount of higher education was capable of doing. Emotions that were not properly nurtured, such as compassion, consideration, understanding and empathy, were now breathing new life within my spirit. Their presence overshadowed any lingering thoughts I might have had of self-preservation. It was a good feeling to not think about myself or my past illness, but instead to be concerned for another. I felt strongly about this, like it was the way I should always live. I wanted to further expand this sense of good in me.

In the months that distanced us from each other, we kept in contact by phone, while she endured what no woman should ever have to. Charlene's voice grew weaker and weaker each time I talked to her. I began to resent the world for allowing this to happen to such a beautiful person. I had a personal stake in this now, and what was happening to her was happening to me as well. I could no longer separate myself from this tragedy. I was beginning to realize that there's no such thing as separateness in human relations. Our fabric is interwoven, and each one of us has the sensitivity of the entire human race. When someone suffers, we all do; when absolute strangers bear burdens of this magnitude, that weight is felt by all in ways we may never know.

Charlene went above and beyond what courtesies I ever thought she would extend me, by taking my phone calls even though she could barely speak. Her pain was severe, yet she talked if even to acknowledge me. She would pause to drip morphine into her mouth with a dropper, while I waited. I just needed to hear her voice one more time. But it was never enough for me, because I knew I was losing her. I thought that if I could hear her, she would never leave me. I tried to hold on to anything I could, that might put off the outcome awaiting her. But a momentum was against us. I remember our freedoms not very long ago when the cup of conversation overflowed and we spilled time as if we had that privilege. Now every word and moment was savored. Charlene's voice was nearly gone. The one thing that bound us from the start was fading. I learned from this never to take things for granted—especially time.

There wasn't much left in Charlene by early December. The few calls I made were answered by Julie. She was decent and tolerant. I don't know how I would've been in her place had I the responsibility to receive so many inquiries while my brother was dying; I just don't know. Nothing was worse than not knowing what was happening to Charlene from day to day, even though I could only imagine.

Some time passed and Julie called me. She invited me to Charlene's apartment for a gathering of friends and family for her sister to see everyone in her final days. I told her that I'd be there. After hanging up, I felt sick to my stomach. I didn't plan on this ever happening, however, I knew this day would eventually come. There was so much to think about; I had so many things going through my mind. My emotions were conflicted in a way that they have never been. I tried to work out in my mind how I might say goodbye to someone forever. What words could I possibly offer that would be enough for Charlene to know what she meant to me? It had been months since I had seen her and I feared I wouldn't recognize her; or worse yet, she would see fear and concern on my face. I wanted to be there to see her; that much I was sure of, so the rest would have to come to me as the moment unfolded.

Would I actually be returning to my past, the same time I was returning to see Charlene? I realized that I was not quite out of the woods myself. My emotional scars had not fully healed, and her imminent fate was hitting close to home. We both were in the same war; I was pardoned by life and Charlene had a death sentence. *How could this be, when she is so much finer than I?* I thought. *Doesn't life see this, that she's so special?*

Just outside Charlene's apartment, the late December winds were vigorous and raw. The sky was overcast; a chilling drizzle dampened

an already somber mood. At times there were brief signs of a struggling sun defiantly breaking through. It was a day common during the
winter months in the northeast. It is the season of endings, when all
that is to be born waits beneath the frozen earth.

I had arrived by plane this time, holding a gift for Charlene. It was
a fully decorated miniature Christmas tree, which stood close to three
feet tall. I wasn't sure what was appropriate for this kind of occasion,
but I wanted to bring something for her. I thought with all that was
going on, Charlene's family might not have had the time or energy to
go out themselves for a tree. I wasn't even sure if they wanted one at
this point. But this was for Charlene.

Katie, Charlene's other sister, was the first to greet me at the door,
with Sophie in her arms. I happened to arrive pretty early; I was the
first guest. Katie went back upstairs to tend to Charlene with Julie and
her mother; I was left with my new pal. There was talk that Katie
would be taking Sophie with her. She was honored to be asked by
Charlene to adopt her most precious commodity.

Charlene was up in her loft where I had never been but always
wondered about. I looked up that way and wondered how she was
doing. I expected to be with company soon and greet Charlene among
them. That's how I thought it would be; it's how I envisioned this
occasion.

I was still removed from a full engagement of Charlene's reality.
Seeing her while in the midst of friends and family would reduce the
possibility of an awkward moment between us. I really didn't want our
last moments together to be in any way regrettable. I would have a
hard time forgiving myself for that. Being with others would provide a
buffer.

Then Charlene changed my destiny with one innocent request.
Julie came down stairs to let me know.

"We're glad to see that you were able to make it, David. It means a
lot to my sister that you came, with the holiday four days away," she

said. "You know, Charlene would like to see you up in her room, if you wouldn't mind."

I will never be able to explain exactly how I felt then and there, at that very moment, and I don't think I will ever try to. But I will say that something kicked in, almost like an adrenaline rush, because I certainly felt that familiar 'fight or flight syndrome,' I used to feel when I played sports in my youth. It was like that and so much more.

I looked at Julie, unfazed, and nodded in acceptance as she went to answer the door. People were beginning to arrive. I saw the stairs just ahead and glanced up there one more time before I began my ascent. I didn't know what to expect. The conflict within me had not yet subsided completely. It would not follow me to her; that I was sure of. Charlene deserved more from me than this.

It was while climbing those stairs that I finally made the decision to tame that hesitant child within. I would take him up into that loft kicking and screaming if I had to. After all, how can I know compassion without feeling deeply, or appreciate life without really living it? This is what it's all about, actually. Nothing else matters but the way we handle ourselves in times like these.

My steps slowed towards the summit of the stairway—catching wind of a smell reminiscent of my time in isolation, many years ago when I too was fighting for my life. It was distinctly familiar yet indescribable. If I had to, I would say that I smelled Charlene's struggle. This briefly brought me back to a time when everything had come to a standstill for me. It brought me back to a place where I had retreated to an inner sanctum, far removed from the hustle and bustle of society. It was soothing. It calmed my fears. It was calming them right then, as well.

My eyes darted around the room in awe of Charlene's fine collection of personal possessions. I noticed the brilliant colors and rich tones of a native Indian rug strewn close by. Antique trinkets were tastefully placed here and there, made by the locals in New Mexico where Charlene lived during her brief remission from cancer. I saw her favorite cowboy boots that were hand crafted in Texas.

Her loft was unusually warm for this time of year, but pleasant and appropriate for the situation. My Christmas tree had preceded me. It perched proudly on an end table by the stairway.

I noticed gentle movement from the corner of my eye, toward the other end of the room, near Charlene's bedside. I stood there waiting to see her, as she sat on a little bench against the wall, eclipsed by her mother and sister, who were still tending to Charlene. As soon as her mother realized that I was there she stepped aside, allowing Charlene to see me.

There she was—the very one I had waited so long to see again. Her eyes were beacons leading me to the shores of her war, as they betrayed her perfect smile that she wore just for me.

I was now in the moment for everything it was worth. It was clear that I could not enter Charlene's world until I had altogether abandoned mine. I was ready to do this.

Her mother offered me an opportunity for privacy. "You probably want some time alone together, so we'll be going downstairs to get things ready for all the arriving guests." I nodded, without a word; I didn't feel a need to respond. It was what I wanted now.

Her mom and Katie walked past me as I closed the gap between Charlene and myself. She had lost more weight since the last time I had seen her, but she was still striking. Stopping just an arm's length away, I took a deep breath and sighed,

"Look at us; once strangers—now friends, and all I can do is look on. You have no idea what this is doing to me." Her brows lifted at center, showing concern. I shook my head in disbelief.

Charlene patted the space next to her, attempting to speak sparingly. "Come sit near me, David."

I could tell that every word spoken was an effort and caused terrible discomfort. I did what she said to do. We barely fit on the vintage wooden bench which brought us much closer to each other than we had expected. Our faces were a breath apart while my legs warmed hers. The early winter sun often peeked through her window between passing clouds; its light not as radiant as other seasons might permit, but was still able to make her short crop of raven-black hair standout most resplendently. Its natural oils were strong, causing her hair to shine lustrously. I was witnessing life resist death right there before me.

I sensed strongly an omen of what was to come in the air, but I never looked away or offered any small talk. The moment was unlike any that I had ever lived before, or might have even remotely imagined would be like. But for some reason I knew exactly what was expected of me, not so much by Charlene, but by life itself. She was forgiving, but I had a feeling that life would not be, had I stumbled awkwardly or influenced the mood.

Charlene's eyes remained poised above her pallid complexion as they carefully searched mine. I saw in them the need for me to commit to the moment, but I already had. I knew how she was in a place no one but I could really relate to. I cared for this woman and I wanted her to know it; I wanted her to know much more than this and I hoped that my being there would be proof of this.

I looked into Charlene's eyes as she looked deeper into mine. The sun once again kissed her face, complementing her creamy—but not rosy—soft skin. Softly, I rubbed her cheek with the back side of my hand, and then gently ran my fingers through her hair while our eyes stayed loyal to each other. It was the first time I had touched her in such a way. I was close enough to her now that I tasted the indelible sweetness of her every breath.

There were no words to fumble with. The moment could not have been more natural. Time stood motionless. It was almost as if it actually waited for us to live out this experience. It set itself aside for us—because of us.

I told Charlene while my eyes steadied hers, that I was there, that it was all right. She knew what I was saying; that I was there in her darkness. She realized that I had been at that same place before, and my eyes were wide open. She was right, I had and they were. I walked this floor before and had seen the very likes of this room. I knew this place; I knew every inch of it.

It was a memory of sorts that I had captured from an earlier time that was mine alone.

All the hesitation completely left me, and I was now in the moment. She knew that I had left my world and was now with her, in hers. I saw this as clear as day in her shining eyes, and will never forget the way Charlene looked at me. She appeared comforted that I would not leave her stranded in this eternal engagement…and she was right; I would have died then and there with her to keep her company. I was devoted to that moment—to her.

Why would I put myself in such a situation as this? I would rather feel momentarily alive with someone dying than forever lifeless among the living. Besides, this was a woman. I had always been taught to sacrifice for them. I had no such echelons of sacrifice to refer to. Sacrifice meant sacrifice. It had no shades of grey that accompany us through life where often the moment's decisiveness is unclear.

Charlene then whispered to me quietly, hoarsely, through a throat that had been ravaged by radiation.

"David, I know a way that I can survive all this. You see, if you let me live through you, a stranger I let into my life and allowed to know me so personally, if you never forget me, then I will truly live past my death. I remember what you once said to me—that when I let you in, I let in the world. You were right; it's what I have always wanted. I think that you've known this of me."

I was flattered that she remembered, but even more, that she never wanted me to forget her. I told her that I've been searching for her longer than she could ever know; and now that I've found her I could never forget her. I've had the thought of someone like her tucked away in my mind as far back as when I first began to anticipate finding that special something that is rare. For a brief moment, Charlene's eyes sparkled with wonder and relief.

We made things right between us; we understood each other.

Charlene's expression showed that she understood more than I did about how this might affect me after she was gone. She didn't want me to be bitter towards life. Selflessly, she asked me not to be resentful for what was about to happen to her. I didn't like making that kind of promise. Charlene knew me; she knew that I would never forget this. *She could ask me anything but that.* I remember thinking.

I was quiet thereafter.

Charlene's pain was becoming unbearable. She searched for her dropper of morphine while grasping gently to her throat. Watching her squeeze the dropper for the numbing liquid was devastating. I told Charlene that I thought she should finish up and prepare herself for the get-together, and that I would get her mother to come up to help her. She closed her eyes and nodded in agreement. And with that I told her that I would see her later on.

On my way down the stairs I was amazed to see the living room full of people. It was such a contrast from where I had just been. I couldn't believe how many people were there to celebrate Charlene's life, to be there for her. The atmosphere seemed appropriately low-key, although anyone who knew better was aware of the deeply solemn mood underneath the thin veneer of pleasantries exchanged.

I lost myself in the crowd by the time Charlene had made her way downstairs with the help of her family. She was in the bathroom with her mother and two sisters, near the entrance door, doing some last minute things that women do, when the airport taxi came to pick me up for my flight. On my way out, I looked to find her, as the door was slightly opened. I could see Charlene sitting with her sisters standing above her. She asked where I was going. I told her the only flight out was leaving and that I had to catch it. She then said to me, in what would be the last words I would ever hear from her, "Will you come and see me again?" I didn't answer her question, but instead smiled, knowing she needed no response.

Four days later, on December 24th, 1994, I received a call from Julie, telling me that Charlene had passed away while in her loft with family by her bedside. Toward the end, they had never left her.

To the question she asked so genuinely about me seeing her again: Of course I will; after all, I never really left her. She is always with me, wherever I am—I visit her memory often. And when I see a beautiful sunrise or its set, I think of her. When I pass a stretch of wildflowers, I envision her lighthearted spirit dancing from one to another. In every woman I meet from there on, I will glimpse a part of Charlene shining through.

I will always remember that day in the loft with a spirited woman who met death with her steady urbane charm, and drifted away into the ages—unconquered.

My sweet Charlene considered what legacy she would be leaving behind. There was no need for this. She will never really know the wake she's created from the ripple of her birth.

I often think about Charlene. I loved her. As I promised during her last days, so will I deliver her to the world—where she rightly belongs.

Be with peace Charlene. All will know of you.

HER CRYSTAL BUFFALO

Often, the greatest beauty to behold
is that which remains forever unfinished.

etters sent to me by Charlene's mother after her death hid revelations that pointed toward her daughter's moral fiber. It had been years since I read them. I missed so much at first in these letters because it was all so fresh to me; I read them as one would—normally. One letter was written several months after Charlene had passed, and the other almost two years later. When I first opened them, Charlene was much more vivid in my mind; her voice was still in my ears. After so much time, to see those letters again brought a surge of remembrance.

I kept them both, along with a wallet-sized picture of Charlene smiling proudly on her motorcycle and a birthday card she sent me in April of 94—with eagerness and expectation for what would be our first get-together—jotted pithily above her endearing signature. It was all that I had of her.

The letters were very important to me because they put into words how Charlene and I related with each other from her mother's perspective. Josephine was able to see this relationship develop. In her writing I found traces of how Charlene really felt about me. I had never known that she anticipated my phone calls. I didn't realize that my voice had cheered her in such a way that her spirit sprang and her heart charmed after our conversations. That meant that I had taken her away from her reality, if only momentarily.

I had forgotten how the words in those letters carried such raw emotion with them from the pen to the paper, by the hand of a mother who had endured an unspeakable loss.

As I read, I felt the past come back to me so vividly. I remembered Charlene clearly, exactly the way that her mother had described her. Each reference to her was able to bridge time as if I could almost see her sassy smile again, as if she had just winked at me so confidently, chasing a remark that had once struck me. I read the letters with a much greater appetite for her than before. I held each page gently, tenderly; like I would hold her, if I could again. I searched every word and between every line for what morsel of meaning I might have missed that would move me the way that she used to.

I found it.

On the second page of the second letter, tucked between a thought of the waste of something so good, and revealing the dreamer of the sisters—that was indeed, Charlene—her mother wrote:

"As Charlene once said to me, when I asked her—openly venting my frustration, 'Why you Charlene?' She would throw it right back to me and say, 'Why not me mom; who would you wish it on? I would rather suffer myself than watch my sisters, friends, or anyone else go through this. What makes me any special?'"

That very attitude made her special. This was Charlene; the person I came to admire.

Is this something humanity can afford to forget or overlook? Are not her words fearless and selfless? From how many lips will we hear such words uttered in a lifetime?

After knowing Charlene, I no longer wonder what it is in a woman that can lead a man to rise to his higher self. Her friendship held all those answers that might've taken me a lifetime to realize.

Charlene's voice still lingers in my memory some ten years later, like the crisp, windswept rustling of the past season's fallen leaves, gathering sporadically here and there alongside an isolated stretch of time. It was what initially bonded us, and what I remember most about her. I suspect time will eventually wipe away even this vestige of her physical presence in my mind. There is nothing I can do about it. There are however, some things beyond time's reach that it can never seize from me, or those who knew Charlene intimately. There are gifts of glory that she left us all in her passing. Each one of us has our own to open, for those who knew her—and of her. Promises of courage and conviction, fortitude and forgiveness, and a never-ending well of fond friendships she's left behind. This is who Charlene was. This is what she has given to us all, and nothing can take this away.

I speak of forgiveness because I've personally witnessed this virtue of hers. It happened when I was with her in the loft, the last time I had seen her. Charlene knew the way that I was; she knew that I would hold life accountable for taking her away from me, from taking her away from humanity. Charlene didn't want me to feel in any way—discontented about what had happened to her. She saw a greater path for me to follow, one of purpose. But what she didn't realize was that these paths would merge. She was right, I've never forgiven life for treating her the way that it did. And even though I'm well aware that this is what she asked of me—to let go of the sadness, and move on—I believe that she was simply being herself, which is much more than I will ever be.

Besides, to forgive certain things not deserving forgiveness would be to overlook a part of her; the part of her that struggled and exposed her greatest attributes, her undying spirit. I'm not willing to do that; not today, tomorrow, or ever. That's the difference between us if ever there was one; I am here to make life accountable for its actions, while she was here to make the world a little more livable, a little more beautiful.

I've always known that my place in this world would be one of duty and dependability. I've known this because life has whispered in my ear thoughts of this nature for as long as I can remember. I felt that one day I would realize the nature of my calling. Even as I talk about forgiveness, a fierce willingness to never forget always remains on the ready. I am not supposed to accept these things without responding to their intrusions, defiantly. What has happened to Charlene was by no means natural and we should never accept this as such. I've seen the truth in that which has taken her way too soon, though I feel even truth at times has no worthy aim.

Nonetheless, each and every year that passes since Charlene's early departure seems to smother what was once a profound passion of mine, now shadowed by so many distractions in my life. Others call it moving on—I have no such intention.

How could I let myself drift so far from the feeling in those letters? I thought. *I won't let that happen again.*

I must nurture these memories that I hold so dear. I must take care to give them attention, as if she was still with me. They will not last on their own, without me remembering.

Watching over the present landscape, I can no longer look on from a distance while I await the approach of those sullen clouds. I know that they will come again, just when we are not ready. There will be another loved one taken from someone's grasp. Our emotions will run a course that can now be predicted by therapists. We will find comfort in company, and those closest to the loss will struggle with it the longest. There will be a point where even their outrage will relent. There will be some, though, who will be duty-bound by this—even empowered.

They will not be able to forget. They will not want to forget. And when they see the truth clearly, they will never forgive until something is done to make things right, till things become natural again.

This will not happen overnight. It will take time and determination, but so many will benefit by this dedication, this devotion to each other—in a much deeper regard.

I have gathered through my hardships and little victories only a handful of memories that have managed to withstand each year with any respectable clarity; memories that give me this inspiration when I need it most. They have proved to be potent. I choose to remember because there is so much to be gained in doing so, and so much to be lost if I don't. I have taken with me all that I've found in Charlene to be admirable. I must take with me the essence of what she symbolized in all women.

You must also see the vulnerability in the hero to know that she was convincingly mortal, conceivable, and emulative. Charlene was no martyr. There was distinction in her character—a duality of sorts, rendering her human. This never kept her from being true to herself; it just made her extraordinary and yet not above adoration. Her virtues were within reach of us all, and this is how she would want it: modest and deliberately confident.

She once spoke of a trip to France that she had taken with her sisters. It was something she had always wanted to do and she saw no reason to forsake a long-held desire. It is a memory of mine that I will never forget. It shows this vulnerability in such a profound way.

It is a stark, lucid scene I have, this vision of a young woman weeping, at times wailing, while kneeling in an archaic French church, as her faith survives barely—in desperate need of resurrection. I can almost hear Charlene gently sob in vain as her voice echoes evocatively throughout the gathering place of souls. All the pews have been abandoned as she noticed herself alone, though we were not what she needed then. It was a moment owned by her alone, however unjust. If she was to find peace in any way it would come to her then, only from within. She spoke to me of the chasm of emotions that overcame her.

"It was liberating!" She declared.

To be able to lash out so passionately, then retreat with humility. Charlene would then laugh at herself while shaking her head in disbelief as she looked to the ceiling in wonder. After exhausting herself, she stared into nowhere, motionless, until tasting one of her tears from the corner of her mouth. She tried to wipe beneath her eyes with her fingers, but the tears had dried themselves. She had lost track of time.

Charlene brought me there with her words. She led me to that private moment for a reason that I may not ever fully understand. But I am so grateful that she did.

As she described the magnificent stained glass, supported by the structure of carved stone that has soundly endured the centuries and even more remarkable—change, I felt whatever stood proudly on that day had been overshadowed by the woman within it—so ardent for life.

Charlene retraced her steps through France's region, but it wasn't long before I was taken back to that same French cathedral. Being in that church meant something to her; she wanted me to see this. It would be the place where I would find her as I've never known her to be. I wanted to know more. I thought: *Please tell me with your voice, that I might soon never hear again, what it was you were thinking—exactly what you were feeling. I'm listening, because you have me—if you only knew how much.*

Charlene's voice held within it the yearning of humanity. Her sorrow was not only hers, just as her sentiments weren't solely of this time. We both were the reflection of many who've lived life just outside of society's numbing effects, at one time or another, and behind our cloaks of individuality, I think we both knew it. Our similar circumstances had caused us to venture far beyond our normal lives and bid farewell to the course we were on. We turned abruptly, then moved toward another way—at different times, but together—whether we wanted to or not. Neither of us would ever be the same again. We were extracting from life much more than we could have ever imagined. We held life in our hands instead of life holding us.

Charlene entered that barren monument alone, stumbling through the unrehearsed. She may have been an individual in search of some sense of reprieve, but the world was with her all along; we all were there.

Charlene, you were never by yourself, not there—not ever. There wasn't a moment when you suffered, that we all didn't. We lived what you lived, wept when you cried, and when you lashed out into the thin air, we heard you Charlene, we definitely heard you. We listened to your voice when it strained ever so much, to share with us those little evidences of life as you lived it. You brought intensity back to me because you confessed to revealing the lesser emotions that over-whelmed you, showing me just how special you really are.

Up in that loft, where a young man and woman met with mutual respect, where two—for a brief moment—became one, we were no more alone than when Charlene knelt in that French church, or when I lay in isolation. Charlene and I were living epically—what so many before us lived through on time's pages; although at that moment it was our stage, it was our theater.

Charlene had found a boutique in France. It was there that she came across a crystal buffalo she just had to have. She brought it home with her because Charlene adored the American buffalo. The buffalo, to her, was majestic. Charlene thought of her crystal buffalo as a symbol of a relation between elegance and strength—wild and refined. She saw the dichotomy in this, but realized even more the pleasing duality. Did she see more in it than I am aware of? That might be. Charlene's vision, at that time, was intensified.

I noticed just recently, in the letters her mother wrote, a reference to her crystal buffalo which was put in a place where all of Charlene's belongings were kept.

Her mother told how Charlene would hold it up to the light and see the most brilliant spectrum of colors. She said that Charlene mentioned how she could see forever through that buffalo. When she saw the light reflect, she got a sense of what is eternal.

A brilliant spectrum of colors, elegance and strength, wild and refined, unbeaten and everlasting—that was Charlene!

It is a rare thing these days to see so much in so little. But when I think back to my days of uncertainty, I remember the statue of the boy with his watermelon and how much that meant to me then. I could actually see once again, my untainted youth. It brought me so much joy. The more that I relate Charlene's story, the more I see how similar our paths really had been.

I remember very well once referring to her statue as a glass buffalo, and her abruptly admonishing me. "Crystal, David, crystal." She affirmed—lightheartedly. I did it mostly to tease her, but now I feel—when I think about what happened to Charlene, that life seems more like glass rather than crystal.

After Charlene died I thought that enough is enough. Of course the medical establishment is legitimate and to be respected, but people are dying anyway—these so called 'legitimate' deaths. No one should be left in the condition Charlene was in toward her end. There's got to be a better way to move forward than continuing the use of treatments that render you physically compromised and unable to fend for yourself at the point when the doctors walk away and send you home to die, telling you and your loved ones that they've done all that they could do. They're right, they have. That's the problem. They can only do so much with the instruments they have at their disposal.

To rely solely upon the doctors can be a very risky adventure. I regard these professionals highly and have no intention of minimizing their efforts, which are admirable. But that doesn't mean that I can't talk about other options and the use of alternative means to complement conventional methods.

Charlene's last days made me realize just how improper our protocol for disease can be.

A time will come when we will look back at this and know that we were approaching disease from a narrow perspective.

My main aim in this book is to bring together the elements of our understanding and merge them—as they should be—as clearly as I am able to, so the individual can walk away with a better picture of how vital it is to first prevent disease by living wholly and attentively, and also to attack disease appropriately if it does come about. When I say living wholly and attentively, I mean that there must be a balance maintained among the relating entities, which I refer to in the chapter so named.

Of course this means that a certain responsibility falls upon each and every individual who wants to maintain good health. There is no other way around this. Like every other living thing that methodically endures through natural instinct, we too must follow higher laws to ensure our survival. Life is not lenient in its rule; it is to be taken seriously.

One need only look to the wild kingdom. There is nothing arbitrary about survival in the wild. In a fundamental way, we are no different. We can neglect our body, mind and spirit to a certain extent because we're resilient, but this cannot be continued for periods of time. The evidence of this limit is all around us in the form of disease, pain and suffering.

I may never know why Charlene, or any woman for that matter, was susceptible to breast cancer. The fact that so many women are afflicted each year is alarming, intolerable and unnatural. It could very well be possible that genetics plays a dominant role in predisposing women to this disease. How far back on the genetic trail this goes is a mystery.

Are we able to thwart its onset? You bet. But first we must be familiar with ourselves in order to know when there is an imbalance. Where to start? Inform yourself. Gain confidence through this awareness. Build from there a strong mind with your will power, with your spirit. When you have accomplished this, you will begin the task of strengthening the body and stimulating the internal systems so they are always balanced and formidable.

Always remember this certainty: the fact that one woman can live through breast cancer opens the gates of life for all women. I cannot overstate this. There are literally hundreds of thousands of women living through breast cancer every year. It is by no means a death sentence. But it is a call to be responsible.

Charlene's circumstance could've gone either way. The most important thing to take with you when referring to her specific situation was that she fought valiantly right to the end. Charlene never gave in; she was a fighter.

Her sisters, Katie and Julie, have Charlene to thank for their lives because they were made aware of susceptibility in their genes by Charlene's diagnosis. This gave them enough early warning to preemptively act upon this knowledge. What they did next would be considered drastic to some, but to others who realize the importance of avoiding breast cancer, this was nothing short of sound judgment. It was done at a time when science was firmly establishing a connection of breast cancer to family genes.

Both Katie and Julie opted to have radical mastectomies followed by reconstructive surgery. This gave them and their families' peace of mind rather than a life of worry. It puts the odds heavily back in their favor.

These are decisions a woman who has this kind of information at her convenience has to make for herself, because it is her life that will be affected by it. They are very tough decisions to make, because of the very nature of them. Julie and Katie saw past vanity; they saw family and life first—their own.

Julie and Katie, in this situation, were pioneers. What they chose may seem to some—unusual, but to me it was nothing less than brave and prudent. Many women will see their courage and find strength to make their own decisions.

Charlene left women hope and strength: hope not in her death but in the way that she defied it.

And strength, showing us that it can come in many forms. She showed women a way to be fearless. Charlene dared to live heroically.

She once asked me why I would want to go through this again, after realizing how close we had become. At first I didn't really have an answer for her because I didn't plan on this happening. But if she was here with me now, she would know that there is nothing I would've rather done than dedicate my time to her. There is nothing I would want more than to be her friend. I wished more than anything else in the world that I could have been on that white horse for her, to have saved her from her fate.

I have hindsight now, and the answer to her inquiry would come to me readily if she were here with me. I would have read to her in my own words the next chapter, because in it shows just what she meant to me, what she gave to me by knowing her, and how she changed my life simply by being herself. Charlene's attraction was inescapable, her influence—life changing.

Even in death her qualities pull me towards her. I'll never forget Charlene; why should I? Why should anyone who knew her? The tenderest part of life exists in memories like these. So, when you hear some say that you should move on and that you shouldn't live in the past, they would only be half right, and their words—a bit lazy. Dwelling on the past has no benefits. It changes nothing; it steals the life away from the present. However, some of the past that defines must go forward with you as you move on. What we have lived makes us who we are. Even more, remembering is the greatest expression of reverence for someone. It's really what we do with the past that matters the most. This takes the best in us to handle it appropriately.

It's easy to get caught up in aphorisms. I've heard many from so many. They seldom impressed me. They seem to neatly package a general truth and require the least amount of thought on someone's part. Life demands a little more from us than to readily accept these phrases. This would be average. Life does not admire average.

Charlene will always be with me. I will take her character, her feisty smirk, her strength, her wit, and everything that she showed me was the best in her. In this way she will be immortal. In this way her fierce fight for life will mean something. In this way her life will survive an early death. In this way will I be a better person for it. My life will be enriched. Remembering the special ones and infusing their traits with yours will undoubtedly make you a better person. That's always a good thing.

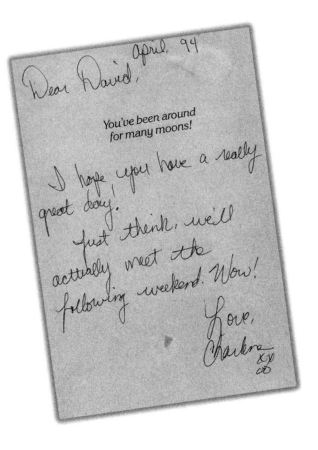

FINDING YOU

The greatest path to finding oneself is often through the spirit of others...the most telling reflection of who we really are.

Charlene was that genuine article I searched for all along. She personified living the way that I wanted to live my life from the day I left that unforgettable room on the third floor of Jane Brown Hospital with nothing more than the barest of life. I didn't have much when I walked away, but inside I was blessed with promise. The best part of me had survived. Life was the spoils of the battle I had just waged. Nothing more than life itself was in my possession, but to me, it was all that I needed. Nothing else mattered.

When California failed to fill an inner emptiness of mine, I realized that I had changed not so much outwardly as I did in how I looked at life. Being normal again didn't have much meaning to me anymore. Normality swallows you up. No one remembers normal for very long. We all remember pathfinders—those who dare to be themselves, regardless of their situation, in spite of how different that may be. We admire this because it is not the easiest path, and it shows an unusual confidence, not so easily had.

I had resigned myself to the fact that I might never feel that way again—so vital for life. In another way, I felt that I was finally beginning to own my past. I no longer felt the need to run from it. My past had so much to do with who I was becoming. It was clear to me that, that which defines you is inescapable. What does free you from the effects of adversity is how you respond to whatever happens in life. There is nothing more important than to have an imposing will through it all. Everything can be overcome when you are with this confidence, when you are with God.

I was home and somewhat settled. My spirit was no longer restless, yet it was far from nourished. It was then that Charlene came into my life, and with her—the renewal of the mystery.

She showed me so clearly how God lives within us all. Our relationship made me realize that religion does not lend us spirituality, but our spirituality is our religion and also our bond with each other. The mystery of that strength—which can heal deeply—holds within it the higher laws of humanity, which reveals the essence of God. I saw this in her. I knew that God was with Charlene. I felt this through my relationship with her. And from the moment she passed, this same essence has never left me.

When I found Charlene, I found the balance that I needed. Purpose showed itself plainly, undoubtedly. That purpose fed my spirituality. That purpose became my religion. That purpose exposed me to God. In this way did I find a religion far above the reach of human interpretation. Charlene freed me. Her life made things make some sense.

If I had the chance to tell her what it was about her that moved me so, I would have to say without hesitating that she gave me the strength to face the unknown, the way I had when I was separated from the world so many years ago.

For a while, before I knew Charlene, I was unsure of my way. Instead of bringing a new way to humanity from what I had gained while alone, society consumed me before I realized what had happened. And before I knew it, I had become ordinary once more.

Knowing Charlene returned me to a place where I had gained my confidence, to a place where there was no room for doubt, our fears, or dithering on matters of great importance. She made me see that what happened to me was not a stigma at all but a precious gift of change, an endowment of empowering transformation. This opened the door to another world, a world I was privileged to live in.

When I was with her in that loft four days before she passed, I was just as close to death as I was in isolation when I was seventeen. I was there, caught within her eyes, ready for anything. If she needed me to die with her right then—I would have. There are things much more important in this world than just surviving. Just ask anyone in their later years if there is any regret for not living passionately or compassionately. Those who are honest will tell you that a lifetime of self-preservation can leave you, in the end, often wanting for peace of mind. I believe this to be true with everything inside of me; that time lived is not nearly as important as the merit of our deeds done while living. It's all a matter of how you want to live, and when you take a moment to think on these very things, you've already begun to welcome the higher laws that can bring you to new heights.

I wonder, in all her imagination, could Charlene possibly have known enough to see, beyond her last breath, all the life she's given back to me? Was she aware that she held the immortal ingredient that I was so desperate for?

She alone showed me what it meant to live vastly in this world, to dare to reach out when it was easier and safer not to. I appreciated and cherished her company more than mere words can express. I can now hold my head high, because I had the honor to walk briefly with a giant and lend comfort to the eyes of a passing angel.

Neither the effects of time nor the distractions of life can ever take that from me. Even when things get tough and my will is tried, I will think of her and I will get through anything. Above all things, Charlene showed me that I mustn't be looking out for myself, but instead I must be in pursuit of need. That is where I will find the greatest rejuvenation of my spirit; it is where I will find my greatest strength—where I will always be with God.

Before Charlene came into my life, I had isolated myself from the world because of vanity and reasons that do not reflect strength, but after knowing her, I learned humility, fearlessness, and a realization that I have so much to offer from what I have lived through. I shouldn't feel separated but should feel a greater responsibility to give back like she did, causing a great wake from a selfless ripple.

If someone were to ask me who Charlene was, I would respectfully respond that she was possibly a sister, a best friend, a close neighbor, a wife, or maybe even someone's mother. In other words, Charlene was a woman...and all that implies. If someone were to ask me who Charlene was to me, I would answer confidently, without hesitation, that she was first a stranger who became my friend, who then saved me, and toward the end opened my eyes to the greatest mystery of all. I'm not afraid of the unknown any longer because I know that she is there, on the other side, just beyond the veil of the unknown—that which shadows the way to immortality.

And wherever you are Charlene, I'm sure glory awaits all those who live the way that you lived.

LITTLE VICTORIES

*Attention to the whole
keeps one modest in all endeavors*

Through it all I feel that I haven't won or lost, I've simply survived. In the course of life's trials there is a sobering realization that victory parades hand in hand with defeat. As it regards to human life, the line discerning the two can be somewhat blurred. When we are with attention, enough to possess a broader perspective, we see that our ups may come during times when others have downs, making our glory somewhat bittersweet; that is, if we are of a mind to experience life with such uncommon sensitivity.

Charlene was not the only significant loss in my lifetime. My father recently succumbed to cancer at the untimely age of sixty-two. By the time I got to his bedside in California—both my brothers there, by him—he was already unconscious. I was unable to show him that I was there; I was unable tell him that I loved him—so that he felt it. He didn't have a chance to see for the last time, his middle son, the one named after him. This was a man who never missed a practice or a game of ours. He would sit in his car for hours while we honed our athletic skills repetitively, day after day. To others this might seem a bit mundane or even a chore, but to my father, this is what he lived for. Every now and then I would look out across the dust and dirt covered field and see him just sitting there inside, or standing—leaning against the fender. I never really thought about the dedication it took to keep such an interest in our progress. Now I know as a man, that to have this in a father was indeed a privilege.

He would pay attention to almost every play, whether it mattered or not. We'd glance up past the grassy hill where his car was parked for the duration of our practice, and he'd always be watching, waving to us in acknowledgment. It was the same for football, then baseball, and for me—wrestling. As we'd fall into the car completely exhausted, he'd recount the events of our performance on the way home. My brother and I fed off of his enthusiasm. It made us want to do even better the next time. I almost thought there were moments that my father lived through us. It made me feel good about myself, that I pleased him this way. There was never any pressure put on us—ever. I don't think that there was ever a time when he ever put us down. There was never a shortage of words of encouragement to be had in his presence.

When the sun was slowly disappearing and the heaviness of the humidity had soaked our uniforms, our faces dripping with muddy sweat, our father would take us for some refreshing local Del's lemonade. Nothing felt better.

That's what I remember. I never told him what this meant to me, to have him care in such a way, to have my father be there for us when he could've been doing almost anything else.

I live with the fact that he never knew how I felt.

I was distracted at that point in my life when he fell ill, and I waited a bit too long to make the trip. It happened so fast. Within months he was gone. I make no excuses, but pledge never again to hesitate when it comes to such serious matters. I have forgiven myself because I know that my father would've wanted me to. I owe so much to him. There were many things I wish I could've told him but I think our trivial differences got in the way. I will never have that opportunity again. Some of our choices can be so permanent. We don't realize this until it's too late.

I have known and heard of many people who've fought fervently for their lives, some have been triumphant and others—unfortunate. I see them all as brave because they dared to defy. They never gave up, even when the pain got in the way of their determination. Humanity inspires me.

We are a defiant people, through and through. More than not I've witnessed strength and perseverance in the character of those whom I've met while in an out of the hospital, and also as we dutifully filed into the clinic for our periodic doses of chemotherapy or radiation.

Those who fight back against death are the most heroic, and even more do I feel this when that struggle leaves them in the end, a better person, one who tends to be selfless. In their hour of darkness, they may reach inward for strength, and that is good, but when they come upon a healing and have ventured beyond the grips of death, they will reach outwardly to others—in their time of need. I wonder if they're truly aware that in this very act of reaching out, they're gaining in ways that cannot easily be measured. What we do on a personal level truly matters.

It's been a long time since my reserves were abundant, as these years I've lived have not shown me relief in the way I imagined that they would. I've taken a tremendous licking physically, emotionally, and spiritually. Still, what I've walked away with I consider immeasurable, and the thought of what I once was could not possibly cause me to regret what's come of me. Where at one time I slept, now I'm fully awake. I'm seeing things that before I could not see, and thinking thoughts I would never conceive of. My awareness has become expansive.

I no longer look at adversity as something I must get past in order to be free or find true peace. Adversity follows me throughout life, as does life's joys. I find freedom from the fear of adversity in the strength and resilience of others. When I see a young woman such as Charlene face the darkness so boldly, few things encourage me more. Few things humble me more.

My victories are little because nothing that I've lived through has been without the influence of others around me. I have been supported. I am alive for this reason.

As a people, we define ourselves by the way we strive and struggle, but do we know that it is in the feat itself that we gather our most sustaining memories? Every cherished memory of ours is defined and validated by our trials and tribulations.

As I reminisce, wanting very much to give to the reader all that I have come away with, I can't help but be reminded that I have been exposed to great humility, which is why every victory of mine I consider to be little. When I look at the big picture, as life has so coarsely shown me, I can't help but be humbled when I see others fight so hard to stay alive and just don't get a break. What I have been through has brought me so much closer to each one of them. When they suffer—I find that I suffer as well. I can't separate myself from this, nor do I want to.

Whether you are privileged or poor, good or bad, compassionate or indifferent, religious or not, no one escapes death. Life's wrath and its natural way is stone cold blind. It is an indiscriminate force that must be understood and not feared, because when we understand it, it has the potential to be very beneficial. In that understanding is found the essence of the higher laws.

Fire is a dangerous, powerful force of nature; it can kill, burn, and cause great pain. When we understand its potential and learn how to make use of it, fire becomes life-sustaining and functional in many ways.

In this way is nature's force to be used—that is, with intelligence guiding each of us.

Sometimes is seems in society there is little interest in the kind of higher laws I refer to. These higher laws have little to do with self-preservation or self-gratification. Maybe this explains the lack of interest.

The higher law's conditions depend upon living in the moment with great attention. A society cannot give this to an individual; it must come from an understanding of life, derived wholly from within. I have not shown different ways to outrun death—it is inevitable. What

I'm suggesting is there are higher laws outside of society's influence that one should become familiar with in order to best prepare oneself for that time when adversity finds you—and it will. What really matters is whether or not this adversity is met with resistance and intelligence.

Will it be enough to take you, or will you be prepared enough to mount a formidable defense? To turn away from the inevitable is a dangerous practice and one that we do often. We just don't think about it until it is at our doorstep. Sometimes by then it is too late. I think this is why there is so much confusion when it comes to coping with adversity, when in fact it does come. We don't want to think about it until it is upon us and then we are desperate for answers in this urgency. We don't know ourselves in the way that we should, and therefore are unaware of our strengths. This is where fear seeps into our spirit, where it has no business being. The only solution for this is having the confidence of knowing oneself according to the higher laws of life.

While there are no small victories in life when it comes to defying death, there is something more to be had in the feeling that when we are victorious from time to time, remembering those who aren't as fortunate should always be in thought. After all, we are in this together.

THE WAY–
NO LONGER ECLIPSED

S o much that happens can shape our lives; so much can provide us direction. These outward influences will always be there to affect us. We have very little control of their presence. In order to know what we should allow to change us and in order to see which direction we should head when we come upon crossroads, there first must be a good sense of self as a foundation. I had the opportunity to know myself in the middle of my losses in a way that ten lifetimes could not show me. A part of me wanted to turn away from change and embed myself in a normal life where I would be safe and comfortable. That's why going to California was so enticing to me.

I gave in to this urge because I didn't have a good sense of myself. The influence that I felt was from within; it was an inner need of the inherent mind which prevailed, because I had no deliberate intention, no higher purpose. You could say that I was set on autopilot. What drove me to seek a normal life was basic. I allowed my inherent mind to get its way without so much as asking myself why I was doing what I was doing. I wonder how many of us really know what guides us through our decisions in life when they aren't really right for us? How many of us are on autopilot? How many of us realize why we are behaving a certain way or desiring certain things? Our inherent mind will impose its instinctual will in our lives if we are not aware. Before you know it, you'll be doing something, going somewhere, or behaving some way that doesn't really make sense or isn't quite rational. Many of us don't realize this until someone brings it to our attention.

When I was in California I lived the way any young man would live. There wasn't a thought about what I had been through. No notion of life was any more profound or enriching than satisfying my basic needs. I entertained relationships that provided intimacy. Women were soothing. Never in my life had I had so much attention than when I was there. And yet, no one could get through to me in a way that meant something, or reach me where it made a difference. I was empty of the most fulfilling aspects of life.

All the time I was satisfying my desires—my most basic needs, there was a deeper deprivation going on within me. I still didn't know who I was; but I was finding out what I wasn't, and that was—normal.

As much as my subconscious desperately wanted this reversal of time, I had grown past it, because I once lived uncommonly; and because of this I could no longer go back to who I used to be. I had awakened an intensity at that time that exists within each of us. It had been roused by necessity. Now it was there, living within me. It was the best in me—original, sincere, and nonconforming. It was doing all that it could to surface and become an imposing force, but I wasn't ready. I didn't listen attentively enough. In a way, I was denying myself.

I had left California understanding that there was so much more to me that I didn't know yet, but I couldn't find it while I was running from myself.

Charlene felt right to me from the moment I first laid eyes on her and heard her thoughts on coping with adversity. The more that I knew her, the more I felt like I was coming home. She was the one who stood me back on my feet, brushed me off, and faced me in the right direction. She did this—and no one else. Charlene reflected what I could not—of myself. She was the doorway to my past. She gave me the strength to see and be who I had become. Through her, I could look back with confidence; something I was unwilling to do on my own. Charlene moved me, mostly without ever knowing. She showed me how natural it was to be whoever we are, no matter what life hands us, to be comfortable with ourselves, even if that makes us unique. She showed me the different faces of beauty. When I met her, I had a semblance of what God was. My spirit was drawing from reserves. I thought that I could go on without spirituality. I didn't know how essential it was to keeping balance within. Charlene's life made me realize my own religion—my spirituality.

In the end, I discovered who I was; I know now what it is that inspires me. I'm no longer conflicted; the best in me has matured into an imposing force which keeps me creative and unafraid. So many have given of themselves so selflessly, to help make me who I am; I feel that I would be letting them down if I didn't own my past. After all, I fought so hard to get through it. And now, my life is deliberate for the first time. The way for me is no longer eclipsed by fear or lack of purpose. I'm not afraid of change. I know that I can handle whatever comes my way. I know this, because I finally know myself.

This whole experience has left such a deep impression on my soul. I will never forget what's brought me closer to knowing myself in a way that one should—really—in a way that one must. What brought me closer to this awareness has also made me want to be closer to others; it's a feeling that's given me relief. That is where I belong. I'm no longer at a crossroads. So much time separates me from my past, but in another way, I'm right back at the beginning, feeling refreshed. My thoughts are pointed in the right direction. My spirit has a full tank of religion to sustain it—this time with my own religion. I'm traveling much leaner than I ever have. I'm focused and the distractions ahead of me will not affect me, only keep me ever aware. I've let go of all that is unnecessary to living purely. I'm trying to keep it simple when I can. I'm unsure what is to come—a concern I have that I feel pales in comparison to knowing without a doubt in my mind where I've been; that knowledge is branded indelibly in my mind.

Even though I lost someone who was able to bridge that gap between myself and the world, someone who made things make more sense to me, I'm able to go on because Charlene's life provided this clarity. I'm confident once again. This kind of confidence is lasting, because it is no longer outwardly conditional; it emanates from deep within.

THE RELATING
ENTITIES OF LIFE

All that defines you reflects
upon nature in the very same manner.

L ife has a definite method of relations between nature, man, and humanity. At all times in our lives an undercurrent of dialogue, harmonious to those aware, chatter to those distracted, is taking place right before us, right within us.

In our quest to understand each part of these relations individually, to control our surroundings to suit us, and possibly to distance ourselves from death's inevitability, we have segregated the entities of this relationship, in affect creating an unnatural division among them. We've lost sight of the entirety of this relationship. We've failed to recognize the interconnectedness of this intricate web of relations between these outward and inward existing systems. Now we are faced with in imbalance of health, and the resulting repercussions of not respecting the intelligence of these higher laws. To further complicate things, we seem to have mystified our natural connections, when in fact, they are simple to understand if we look at it sensibly.

There exists a great force of intelligence to which every living thing is connected to this vital energy. There is nothing more powerful or omnipotent than this healing force. Call it God or what you will, just be aware of it because it is there. It is part of nature. We are the reflection of nature, and in that reflection we have within each of us a balance of relating entities as well. This is because we are no different than nature, but are the manifestation of nature itself, and that is why we are sensitive to what happens around us. That is why we must understand who we are individually in order to relate to nature and humanity in a healthy and appropriate way.

We cannot bully our way through life awkwardly, without consideration for these principles. This will get us nowhere. We must move through life with grace and virtue guiding our actions. Because in the end, what we do to nature we do to humanity, and what humanity does collectively affects each one of us right down to a cellular level. We cannot avoid each other or create distance from our actions; we are inescapably bound. This inquiry into who we are is not one of self-gratification; we are only seeking individuality in this way to be at our best for the greater good of humanity. Each individual link is vital to the chain, but the chain cannot strengthen the link, although it relies completely on each link for its strength; whereas, the individual link is responsible for its own strength. So then, the individual link brings to the chain its strength, but must acquire its strength inherently from within. Every one of us must assume this responsibility.

So what is it that bonds us with humanity so intimately, and what is it which unites humanity with nature in an ongoing dance of life?

Enter the relating entities.

These are the entities which comprise the basis of this very interaction between man, humanity and nature. There is the total mind, consisting of the creative and inherent mind—respectively; both are indefinable to the human senses. In other words, their existence cannot be touched, seen, heard, or in any way realized except by the mind itself, which may be intuitive.

In a well balanced individual, these joint entities are operating as one, as they should be; although, the creative mind must govern the inherent mind for there to be a proper relationship, to be freed from instinct and the primitive emotions.

We see this as an interaction between the internal systems—both voluntarily and involuntary, and an external interaction between man, humanity and nature. Thus we have the existence of a creative and inherent mind which concertedly coordinates this ongoing process throughout the life of the individual. The balance of this finely tuned phenomenon is further sustained by the human spirit or the will of the people.

In that very capacity exists the intelligence and creativity of the universe—literally at our fingertips.

When it comes to the creative and inherent mind, one cannot survive in a healthy condition without the other; they co-exist. The creative mind has within its reach the comprehension of the higher laws. The inherent mind has the knowledge of humanity along with the instinctual intelligence—of all that has been and is here and now. Together, with the spirit guiding both, they can accomplish the unimaginable. We are nowhere near utilizing our capability, but are finally realizing that we are most capable if we can only get past the marvel of this potential and apply our understanding in our everyday lives. We must believe in ourselves; we must believe in each other.

It is important, however, to keep in mind that centering ourselves is what we're aiming for here, along with attaining a certain comprehension of how things work and relate to each other. The goal is to avoid losing sight of the main objective, which is realizing just how much we are in control of our faculties, and ultimately what happens to us regarding our health. I have an obligation to stay on this course, to achieve this very purpose, even though it's easy to digress when explaining subjects as complicated as this one can be. But if I can understand this, there is no reason why anyone can't.

The brain and the body are tangible entities, physical in nature, so they are inescapably subject to a certain set of rules defined by the science of nature, thus submitting to the properties of its laws. Although these laws are arguably bendable, nonetheless, they are still held undeniably within the limits of them. This makes the brain and body vulnerable without the guidance from the intangible entities—the creative/inherent mind—where is found the elusive spirit, our bond with the intelligent vital force that courses through us when we are confident and balanced.

The human spirit, however, has its own vast infinite threshold which we are only just beginning to comprehend. It is where I believe all of the potential of healing resides. It is my contention that the mind is only the means for the spirit to influence the body. The mind alone is like a force without direction, leaving intelligence, creativity, imagination, and inspiration—still. The spirit ignites the creative/inherent mind. It is the hidden hand which allows the greatest mystery to enter into the mind, making all possible, all achievable.

The brain is the physical control center of the central nervous system, which is the trigger to the endocrine system, which in turn stimulates the all-important immune system; all of which depend upon the influence of the creative/inherent mind for proper function. Without the human spirit continually persuading the creative/inherent mind, through thought, desire, will, and a wide range of emotions, the physical self remains motionless, and eventually tilts out of balance; at which point a vulnerability to the forces of nature presents itself, and we are at once exposed to the whim of circumstance, and a host of opportunistic organisms waiting to impose their will on us. If we are not imposing our will then there will be an imposition against us. It is the way of life.

The body, being physical and therefore limited in its strengths, is the only setting for our spirit to reach out to others in so many important ways that can be both sustaining and maintaining in another balance of individuality *and* reliance among the living systems. It is an ebb and flow of give and take between these systems. It is in this way that we begin to see the need for all relating entities within the self, to be healthy, balanced and in harmony, in order to interact with others appropriately and beneficially. But even more imperative is the necessity to understand, to know that that which holds the greatest potential of all is captured within the human spirit. Without this understanding of who we are and how we relate within and without, the whole interaction would eventually misfire and in time break down.

We must be in control of our internal living systems. If we look at each of the entities and understand their function as they relate to each other, we will see that there is clearly a balance of responsibility which must be respected, in order to maintain overall health. Health does not just happen; we must provide the environment for it to thrive. This falls upon each one us because we are free. In that freedom there are conditions. When they are respected, health is ours.

As I've said earlier, what is internal is a reflection of that which is external. What goes on within us very much resembles what goes on in humanity and in nature. I'll further explain this when we've better understood what we share within us all, as I define the relating entities.

We've now been introduced to the creative/inherent mind, of which volumes could be written about. Put simply, the creative mind should be, when all things are in balance, the governing entity of the inherent mind. It is also where the will or the human spirit should prevail, even though it flows freely to and fro—between the creative/inherent mind. The actual brain, being physical in nature, is where these entities perform day in and day out. Their duties leave traces for us to see, in the way of impulses, energies and all sorts of brain activity which can be very interesting for the scientist, but not nearly as revealing as is accomplished routinely on any given day, by the creative/inherent mind and the human spirit, as a whole.

The inherent mind—the instinctual and intuitive side of the total intangible mind—is the storehouse of our personal experiences. It is where our genetic disposition —including character tendencies, inclinations of response to external relations and the collective knowledge of humanity and its history exists. It is the auto-pilot called upon by the creative mind during times when the creative mind retreats, submits or is any way distracted by vital emergencies of the moment. During these times, the inherent mind operates predominately the motor skills of the individual. It is responsible for the function of the autonomic nervous system—the immune system, breathing, circulation, digestion, metabolism and hormonal balance. It does many of the things performed without the attention of the creative mind. In the meantime it continually regulates all the involuntary functions of the body.

If we look further into the inherent mind and its place among the relating entities, we see that, first and foremost, it is the remnants of our once dominant instinctual mind. We, at one period in our evolutionary timeline, relied upon it exclusively, long before we liberated ourselves through self-awareness. The inherent mind is older and significantly more methodical and predictive than the creative mind.

The creative mind, on the other hand, is a new born and has only recently been liberated from the inherent mind, in that it has allowed the individual to realize existence and also to evolve in ways never before imagined. The inherent mind still performs almost exclusively the tasks in the body. The creative mind still relies heavily upon the inherent mind for this, although I believe in time, through evolution and intelligence, the creative mind will dominate the inherent mind in these actions as well. The creative mind will slowly realize its abilities and will intervene when necessary, to influence many functions that are now the sole responsibility of the inherent mind.

This will take a disciplined mind. We see this on a small scale in individuals who accomplish amazing feats. Another book could be written on these stories of extraordinary abilities, but we have all been privileged to this knowledge, enough to know that it is real. We know that there are people who achieve what was once thought impossible. It happens every day. I believe that if one can, all can. I've always believed this.

For now however, we must negotiate our influence over the inherent mind because it still has the upper hand of seniority. The inherent mind acts out of basic emotions and because of this, the creative mind tempers the responses of the inherent mind through logic, understanding, reason, rationality, and the higher laws—all attributes of the creative mind. The creative mind holds so much potential yet to be realized—yet to be utilized. This is simply a matter of patience, discipline and understanding.

Within the inherent mind are the experiences of humanity's distant past and of the individual's recent past. These impressions interact with one another and give birth to tendencies, perceptions and interpretations of truth as seen through the eyes of the individual. We become prone to react in a particular way, to a particular situation, or stimulus, depending upon the tendencies in our inherent mind. The effects of these tendencies determine our character. We respond to situations in differing ways, according to the character of the individual and the way the individual perceives and interprets his or her surroundings. With this realized, it must be noted that the inherent mind, being instinctual in nature, responds to its environment involuntarily, with a somewhat skewed view of the world, an overly protective view I might add.

It is self-preserving and crude in its emotions, having basically one goal—survival. It resists change in any way, because change brings the unknown; and in the unknown awaits possible death. It seldom lives in the moment but instead secures itself in the past and fears the future. The inherent mind is very uncomfortable with unpredictability. It is similar to a defiant child in that it needs to be structured and reassured by a confident, creative mind and a vital, imposing spirit.

When the inherent mind is in control of the total mind, the individual tends to live in the past and react to life through preconceptions and inappropriate interpretations to the present moment. The inherent mind is also very reactive to outside stimuli and much less prone to see the truth of a circumstance. This puts the individual at odds with reality.

The inherent mind uses the collective experiences of the past to protect itself; the creative mind draws from this knowledge to better relate to the world. When the inherent mind is dominant, the child acts out, but when the creative mind governs the inherent mind, which happens when there is confidence, then the child within reaches out in wonder and reassurance.

The inherent mind is to a certain extent self-centered, but it can also be destructive when it gives hidden messages of having little self-worth or being undeserving of life's beauty. I believe it does this in order to bring the creative mind into submission, so that the creative mind does not create change. It would, if it could, swallow the creativeness of the creative mind, just so that it could remain with routine, patterns of predictability.

The creative mind is new in evolutionary terms. It is the voluntary side of the intangible mind. It is the individual's clean slate, a blank canvas waiting for the human spirit to paint its masterpiece. It has the potential to be what you bring in the way of creativity to humanity. It is your means of contribution to mankind. The inherent mind ties us to the past. The creative mind provides a self-evolving promise for the future. Together they perform in harmony right here in the present.

The creative mind lives in the moment and is in touch with the higher laws. It understands the importance of living the higher laws and implements them. The creative mind is self transcending. It adapts itself and is self-evolving. The human spirit influences the creative mind and is spiritual.

The human spirit is the connection between the vital life force of intelligence and the creative/inherent mind. It is a religion that unites and bonds humanity; it is transcending in this way as well. The human spirit centers the creative/inherent mind. The human spirit and the creative mind are in tune with the higher laws while the inherent mind still follows the laws of nature which are solely instinctual.

Out of the three ego states, the adult ego state defines the creative mind the best, while the parent and the child ego states share both sides of the mind, depending upon the maturity and balance of the total mind. When the creative mind understands that there is no permanence in life, and therefore refrains from accumulating possessions, thoughts, knowledge, or anything that suggests to the inherent mind a fear of loss, then the inherent mind is at once freed of this fear and the intelligence of the great mystery is allowed into this sacred ground, where the vital force of life flows unimpeded throughout the living system.

It is very important to spend your life developing your creative mind because that which is mostly involuntary is within reach of the creative mind. There will be a time when the creative mind will eventually influence the involuntary functions of the body to the point where we will be able to affect our health directly by imposing our will upon ourselves internally. It is absolutely being accomplished in the here and now, but not with any consistency. Presently, our ability to alter our health by way of the creative mind is more a hit or miss effort. The human spirit is of course the key to ultimately accomplishing this, but again, there are many aspects of this that must be implemented before any substantial ground can be gained.

The creative/inherent mind is vital to the balance of the relating entities. In order for this, the total mind must itself be balanced and in constant dialogue with each other, along with having a strong influence from the human spirit. An example of this balance is when we are driving; the creative mind is at times distracted in thought when it really should be focused on the immediate task of driving. The inherent mind is right there to act as autopilot until the creative mind realizes it has been away from attention to the moment, hopefully before being wrapped around a tree. In this case the inherent mind stepped in on the creative mind when it was needed.

Or consider when we are asleep and the inherent mind is caught in a nightmare which brings anxiety and fear. The creative mind still very much aware, enters the dream, giving the message that it is only a dream and not real, and then it proceeds to abruptly bring an end to it. This provides us with the knowledge that the creative/inherent mind share responsibilities, acting almost as one—continually.

To have this type of balance brings confidence to the living system on a level that escapes our consciousness. But there is no doubt that our bodies are listening to this relation.

Every cell in our body takes direction from something, with the unity and unison like that we see in a school of fish or a flock of birds; each moving like the other, swift and instantaneous. It is a great force of wonder and awe. So where exists the will—the spirit of this army of cells? Where is the leader, or better—this command center? It lives within the brain, the central nervous system, and the immune system, where it is most powerful and useful to the body. The brain floats suspended in a brine of electrical ebbs and flows, awaiting its master's direction, like a great ship at sea ready to set a course for the uncharted and vast horizon. The human spirit is at its helm, whether or not it is a leader is of the utmost importance, especially when it comes upon troubled waters.

Envision if you will, your body composed of a large army of soldiers. A chain of command leads to one leader who gives the orders, one who ultimately directs. The army of soldiers obeys this direction. The cells in your body are this army of soldiers poised to respond at a moment's notice. But like any army, they must respect their leader in order to perform with purpose, loyalty and dedication. They must sense within the body a deep confidence. This can only come about when there is balance and unity among the relating entities. It is the goal of the individual to be aware of this balance and know what it means to achieve it at all cost. The health of the individual depends upon it.

There is freedom composed of words and notions of such, but few of us know really what it is to be free. The most significant freedom is reached when the creative mind and the inherent mind are no longer conflicted, when the myths that haunt the inherent mind are dispelled. As of yet, we are still—to a great extent—under the influence of the inherent mind.

One of the great conflicts which must be settled in order to create harmony between the relating entities within is to still the inherent mind. The inherent mind must be prevented from seeking distractions. It must see the moment for what it is, not to hold onto it, but see it and then release it, so that it is ready and aware of what is next to come. This way, it is not caught in the past, but instead it is with the creative mind, working as one, in the present.

The inherent mind likes to dig deep into its memory. It prefers to compare, interpret, and perceive reality according to what it already knows. It wants to prove again and again this continuity of what it believes to be true. You must see to it that it does not do this. That is why it is important to be imposing; it is important to live in the moment with vitality. This will keep the inherent mind at your command. The creative mind must always occupy the territory of the part of the mind that wanders. Either the creative mind is dominant or the inherent mind will run wild. The inherent mind is a very powerful entity that wants what it wants. Instinct drives it. The creative mind has the responsibility to manipulate this force, to do what it is supposed to do—for the creative mind, for the individual. This is how we've evolved. We cannot turn back this evolution; we must go forward. We must assume control; this takes maturity and inner strength.

True freedom is an individual endeavor. No words can bring to you this freedom. No other can afford you it. But once it is secured, you will realize what it means to be free; free from the fears, the myths, the past, distractions from truth, and from the influence of the inherent mind.

EMOTIONS
THAT WITHER

*Where thoughts venture, and what
emotions prevail, the body is not far behind.*

L ife certainly has intent, but its intent is not driven by malice or mercy. It took me a very long time to see the truth of this. We give life human characteristics through our perceptions and misunderstanding. When I realized this, I began discovering that I had much more influence over my circumstances than I had previously thought. I was also learning that there are rudimentary emotions fixed within our basic design that affect important functions in the body. These are primitive emotions which exist at the very core of survival; I refer to them as passionate response emotions. Handled properly, these emotions are appropriate and a necessary part of inward and outward relationships of living systems.

Through perception of a truth or a situation, whether it is past, present, or what is to come, we have triggers for actions and responses. We are stimulated by what we perceive as a reality, whether or not it is actual. All of the senses contribute to this stimulus, even the sixth sense. The mind interprets this information through receptors which channel these impulses to the central nervous system. From there the responses begin.

The autonomic and peripheral extensions of the central nervous system that are biologically connected to the endocrine and immune system, signal to appropriate glands for the release of hormones specific to the needs of the proper response to the stimuli. In turn they activate certain processes throughout these internal systems that— depending on the duration of this stimulus—may or may not benefit the overall health of the individual.

Fortunately, we don't have to delve too deep into science to extract that which is most useful to us. All we need do is scratch the surface of this remarkable chain of events which instantly takes place within the body. We have to realize that what we perceive and the way we interpret our circumstances from moment to moment directly affects us physiologically. This can either work for or against us, depending on our ability to direct our minds, and be without presumptions.

There is a well of thoughts and memories deep within our center of many experiences from the past and apprehension toward the future. These thoughts and memories tend to have our attention while we are awake and asleep. They can take us out of the present, where we should always be. Memories have a way of evoking emotions and intense feelings vividly, as if they had just happened. If we're not careful to moderate our thoughts, they will overwhelm our ability to be productive in our everyday ventures, and see life in the now—as it really is. Remembrance is an essential part of interrelations, and also an indispensable means for survival—in its place, of course. Thought provokes; it inspires—if it is right thought.

The inherent mind, which is all that we have lived and what humanity has given to us by way of memory, genetic imprint and intangible tendencies, harbors the encounters of the past, like a great storehouse of information.

Within these past experiences contain our personal history, what has happened to us while we are alive, and, the collective history of civilization, which is the accumulation of life lived, throughout the centuries. They are ours by way of inheritance, and we are subject to their influence, on a physical, emotional, and, many times, spiritual level.

Through time, we have evolved into free-thinking people, with the ability to overrule our instinctual mind; and in that progression we have gained proudly, albeit far from mastered, the capacity to separate ourselves from the animal world. This enables us to manipulate our attitude towards certain situations. We have the ability to choose the way we interpret what happens to us, through thought and attention, reason and logic. We have the ability to respond to our environment appropriately. In the realm of disease, the ability to master one's emotions reigns supreme when it comes to coping with the uncertainty of illness. At no other time in our lives do our emotions become so significant, as when our health fails.

The freedom to influence the central nervous system is still an undeveloped and evolving means. If we misapply this newly acquired control, it can also work against us; that is, if we haven't perceived our surroundings according to reality, but more as a result of prejudices, beliefs, fear, insecurities, and so on—which have been brought to the surface by the inherent mind. The inherent mind influences our perception when we haven't a clear understanding of reality. The creative mind, a part of the mind which interacts with reality in the now, voluntarily, must always be at the helm for proper direction of the body and whole mind to exist in harmony. The inherent mind is fascinating in its ability to react to the creative mind, while at the same time executing extraordinary tasks within the body. The inherent mind performs all the necessary responses that range from alerting the creative mind of any imbalance within the living organism with "gut feelings", to monitoring proper functions of every inner system; it does this involuntarily. This is our instinctual intelligence. But when left to react to the moment on its own, without some guidance, its response will be drawn from our basic human emotions, and its reactions will reflect this.

The creative mind is guided by the higher laws; virtuous laws that are above the rudimentary emotions.

When the inherent mind is calm, without fear, and guided by the creative mind, it is as free as the creative mind. They become one, seeing as one, listening as one, contemplating as one, creating as one, and so on; as this happens, the energy of life flows through every cell in the body, replenishing reserves and aligning with all that lives. The creative mind and inherent mind should share every moment by continually interacting in perfect unison, with no resistance or inner conflict to impede the flow of the healing force. When the mind is performing properly and appropriately and without inner conflict, there will cease to be outer conflict; this will bring health to the individual.

There are many ways for thoughts, emotions, and actions to wither our life force and further bring inward and outward imbalance among these relating entities we have recently discussed in depth. Repressed, destructive, emotions—unresolved—are stresses on the body that continually suppress the immune system and lead to the manifestation of many diseases.

There is an emotional cancer to be aware of. It can be just as deadly as cancer itself. This cancer of emotions slowly eats away at your creativeness, your confidence, and ultimately, your spirit. It happens when you are not master over your thoughts and emotions. Like cancer, these malignant thoughts and emotions smother healthy ones, overwhelming the mind.

We can distract ourselves from unhealthy thoughts and harmful emotions for a while, but to do this is a temporary fix. Suppression will not make them go away. Our true strength lies in our ability to first understand, then confront our most deep rooted fears and concerns, bring them to light, and see that they are not worthy of controlling our lives. There are clear and decisive ways to do this that require realizing self-worth, recognizing pure innocence, abandoning the weight of the past, and learning the art forgiveness. These can be extremely potent neutralizers to the perceptions that wither our spirit.

One of the first things that I noticed had changed in me after losing my best friend to a trauma-induced memory loss was my emotional balance and attitude of confidence. Hope and contentment had abandoned me; guilt, despair, fear and doubt had replaced them. Apathy came over me. I felt at times that I didn't deserve to live. I punished myself for the accident we were in, and never knew how dangerous it was to be without pardon. I couldn't predict how unforgiving life would be toward me for holding these self-destructive thoughts for too long; but I soon found out. I was diagnosed with a type of cancer where the body attacks itself. I was beating myself up internally; the game I was playing had become a serious one.

I learned from that experience how, without question, emotions play an important part in illness—possibly the lead role. Interactions between internal systems within my body were taking place. Functions of the immune system and the central nervous system had been affected directly by my thoughts and emotions. This was much more than theory; it played out in real life.

I had heard many times that a positive attitude can help one through many things, but to me that was always a vague notion. It sounded like hope without action, which to me was weak. It's the emergence of a dream that, without being pursued, will never reach fruition. There had to be action involved, connecting hope with health. I began to realize the significance of my input to bring the two together.

What I had learned actually put that theory into motion. It made sense now; it was something I could believe, because I lived it firsthand.

But was it a stretch to think that my emotional state set the stage for this tragedy? Was I ready to accept this kind of control and responsibility; and if so, in what way? So many more questions crossed my mind. The moment I could answer one, another would surface.

Interestingly, the questions came with a sense of order to them, like I had discovered a secret message that had already been there but was not yet noticed. Once I was able to see this, the answers came to me like a gentle breeze let into my mind from the vast immenseness of a great mystery. If I wasn't careful to know this when it came to me, it would be gone in an instant, without so much as a trace of its presence. I think this is how it escapes most of us. It doesn't come to us in any grand way, but instead gently nudges our senses while we're busy living, or more the case, being distracted. Attention is the key here. It's a great waste to not be aware. But if we were aware, we might realize something omnipresent, and then this awareness would never leaves us.

It took some years for it all to come together, but time wasn't an issue; I had plenty of that. Ever slowly, life showed me what I was missing. I learned how there are many emotions and thoughts that can wither our spirit, and how this happens in so many ways. I realized how weeds that sprout from these seeds in our minds steal the water from the beautiful thoughts—secretly sapping their life force. If gone unchallenged, eventually such weeds will overtake the garden. Emotions like fear, doubt, jealousy, anger, hate and selfishness, wither our spirit, causing us to slowly lose heart, and also our way in life. Feelings of hopelessness, futility, and lack of purpose, degrade our morality, further draining the healing energy. It doesn't have to be constant, just consistent. Not only do these unhealthy seeds sprout weeds that manifest outwardly toward others around us, but these seeds grow roots that affect our inner balance as well. The deeper these roots are allowed to grow the harder they are to get rid of. Just as weeds in nature need nourishment to grow, so do these types of roots need attention for their sustenance, as well. This attention can come in many forms, but ultimately, it tends to take away from the attention of the moment, which is where the healing energy exists.

All of this is likely to oppress the best in us, and then we are not benefiting from the higher laws. Ultimately, we are not with God.

These emotions have survived death's threshold by way of our inherent mind. Many times our perception of circumstance is influenced by the inherent mind in subtle ways. As said previously, the inherent mind acts on fundamental emotions, while the creative mind is rational and reasons, but all too often we rely on the inherent mind for our responses to life, and this is where there is conflict; because the inherent mind cannot distinguish reality, so it draws from its memory, from the most basic of human emotions.

Some of these memories of emotions are not healthy responses to reality, but they've been passed down through generations and are as deadly as any poison can be. Society has a force of its own that's filled with chaos, security, imitation and redundancy. In society's way there can be a very negative force. It thrives in the realm of confusion and self preservation.

This is real and relevant to health, as my personal experience points to. I must learn all that I can about these connections between the central nervous system, the immune system, the total mind, the human spirit, the past and present. I need to find out how these separate things interact with each other to bring about change within us, and where it is the healing energy comes from. Can it be found in society's way, or is it only the shadow of this energy that we're familiar with? Must we then find it—alone?

There are thoughts in our minds that wither, just as there are those that are capable of great promise and beauty. Is my perception of life the puppet master of my emotions? Am I the one really in control of my destiny, or am I fooling myself into thinking that I am? Can I break free of the past and all of its conditioning on my belief system, so that I might finally realize this true freedom that I have stumbled upon during my recovery? Has the healing force been within me all along but I was too distracted to draw from it— to inherit it?

It stands to reason then, that if thoughts and emotions can wither and leave us vulnerable, they can also sustain, rejuvenate, and protect us from harm.

There exists the actual, and, too, the shadow of the healing force. One is God and the other is the interpretation of God in society.

There is the idea of what we want God to be, and then there is what God is. Here lies a part of the conflict within us that we struggle with, on many different levels of being; what we want to be, and what is.

We form our interpretation of this mystery we think of as God, to somehow try to control and manipulate our surroundings in our effort to be safe from circumstance and provide permanence in a temporal life. But is this not a distraction from life itself, this deception? If we seek security in an insecure world, how can we ever know the truth of healing when the truth is alive and flowing in the moment; and the moment is anything but secure? Unfortunately I don't think we can have it both ways. Security does not exist in nature. Mind-sheltering from threat is no safer than facing it head on and prepared. In fact, the more we seek this form of refuge and safety in the known, the weaker our resolve becomes, and the further we distance ourselves from the healing energy. Life to me is either a brave endeavor or meaningless. We are either in the game, or we are only spectators waiting for death to come to us.

In the past, by not understanding these higher laws, I allowed myself to be within harm's way, within the reach of society's influence. This left me with feelings of guilt, fear and doubt that society's tradition had handed down to me without question, without regard. In doing so, I was left vulnerable to circumstance.

Without a master at the helm, a clear sense of direction or inner confidence, the internal systems within my body, which are responsive, such as my immune system and the central nervous system, shut down or turned on itself. I believe this happened to me because I abandoned my command post. I lost my ability to be imposing; and in doing so I lost my way. I unknowingly was letting thoughts of guilt take root in my mind. I blamed myself directly for my friend's condition—for the accident. I became my own judge and jury.

This allowed circumstance to take over and alter my destiny. How many of us have sabotaged our health in ways we try not to admit, or hadn't occurred to us, until now? Think about all the ways that we can affect our health through surrendering to vice, giving in to our own negative thoughts, and expressing inwardly and outwardly, emotions that wither our spirit. Think about what this does to us when we carry this weight on our shoulders. How can we know what true freedom is when we're chained to the past by so many memories of being slighted in some way that we can never seem to get over? How can life be passionate, as it should be, when we are with these destructive thoughts and memories?

Forgiving myself for the accident came way too late for me. How many of us are inviting death to our door without knowing it?

Cancer comes in many forms, with many different reasons why it manifests. The dynamics are intimately intricate and involving, with uncertainties beyond our control. That doesn't mean that we cannot overcome. What it does mean is that cancer becomes formidable when we are not with truth—not with the healing energy. Cancer comes to us when we are not paying attention. It comes when we are waiting and not doing.

We've looked at what can put us in harm's way if we're not careful with our thoughts, if we entertain for too long—emotions that wither. We've seen firsthand how one can be vulnerable to a life threatening disease by way of perception and interpretation. We also know that we have much more control over our situation than we might've imagined. We know now that we can be imposing; we can take action. Let's look at what it takes to really be confident, balanced and self-empowered. Let's look further inward to examine our true strengths. Let's see what we require for us to be imposing.

THE ESSENTIALS
FOR AN IMPOSING
CREATIVE MIND

When you want health, you must ready for disease.

Not only is there to be all-out confrontation with cancer physically, in the way of nutrition, proper rest, deliberate healing movements, and when appropriate—seclusion, but even more important, in my eyes, is the psychological and spiritual engagement that must be realized within the individual. There should not be the slightest hint of doubt, or thoughts of retreat anywhere within the creative mind. Above all, it must be committed to maintaining hope in the spirit. It is only then that one will have a life force capable of imposing itself against such a threat to survival as cancer has proved to be.

The creative mind is the governing entity in the balance of relations within. That's a big job.

The inherent mind, no less important, is a step behind—ready and waiting to respond to the messages delivered from moment to moment by the creative mind; this, by way of thoughts and emotions influenced by the human spirit, that reigns over all entities within. The human spirit is the essence of the total mind's relation with the life force which flows through every living thing and every individual cell in the body. The higher laws in life are what keep one within reach of this immense intelligence. There can be no overly dramatic description of the human spirit. It is a direct reflection of the great mystery, holding within its grasp the promise of an unfathomable inner strength that one can only really know when living in the moment.

When the creative mind is focused in the present, clear of all distractions such as fear, doubt, anxiety, or any other self-defeating emotion or thought, it performs flawlessly. In this state, it is "in the zone".

There is much to be said about this place we call the zone. It is real. When it is experienced, you cannot be distracted. You are in a place where no one can interrupt you. You are balanced, focused, and do become a force to be reckoned with. Life's force is flowing through you unimpeded; and all of your senses—including the sixth sense—are keen and attentive. Your objective is clear. You can see past your adversity, and you find a way to get there. I cannot benefit from the intelligence of life's vital force unless my creative mind is formidable. It must be imposing, sure of itself, directed, inspired, liberated, and attentive.

The creative mind should resist any conformity to outside beliefs or opinions that it has not completely accepted after careful consideration. Conversely, it should not relinquish authority to the inherent mind, because the inherent mind is very suggestible, and will accept anything allowed to bypass the creative mind. The inherent mind does not operate with logic; it hasn't the ability to reason, so the creative mind must be ready for this. The inherent mind must be guarded by the creative mind because this portion of the mind is the entryway to the inner sanctuary of the body—with all of the meaning that this implies.

That is why it is so important to know yourself. By having this familiarity you will gain confidence. And confidence is a state of mind that is essential to balancing the body, mind, and spirit, so that all work together in harmony.

What then are the characteristics of an imposing creative mind? How does one know that his mind is in proper balance in regards to these relating entities within? Let's look at some traits of a survivor such as me. I cannot speak about what is in the minds of others but I know very well what defines me. When I have come across stories of survival, I see again and again an underlying theme. Like me, survivors find a way through adversity no matter what; to them there is no other option but to push ahead. They realize what is at stake and accept their life as their own responsibility.

Survivors are self-motivated and self-initiating, because they know that creativity is a part of self-reliance. There's nothing more moving than being inspired, but when there's no inspiration around to be had, then a back-up plan is the next best thing, and a survivor realizes this. When it comes down to it, this is your life; no one can save you from death if you are not right there on the front line of defense. If you're only a spectator in your recovery, than all the support in the world may not be enough to save you.

Support is fine and needed, as we all seek comfort in this way, but it will not always be there when you need it. Life promises something much more dependable to everyone.

I have met many people who have lived through cancer and adversity, alike. I found their attitudes about their ordeals compelling and inspirational. There was always a resounding theme. It remained there, between each different account; within the many stories told by these survivors was a truth that defined every one of them similarly. I've gathered some common characteristics among survivors that I thought was worth noting, so that you can see what seems to succeed when fighting for one's life.

SURVIVORS—

- never feel helpless under any circumstance
- feel that there is always an option yet to be discovered and will spend as long as it takes uncovering it
- will pick themselves up when the chips are down, and become their own pep squad

- tend not to resent or harbor ill feelings for very long; and they also know how to let things go
- do not deal with things by being in a state of denial; a survivor prefers to know the reality of a situation rather than being kept in the dark
- are stubborn right to the end, in that they refuse to give up or give in
- take an active part of their own therapy
- welcome change while keeping a guarded mind
- are spiritual in a very personal way
- know how to express themselves, and aren't afraid to show it
- are committed to doing whatever it takes to recover
- are passionate about life
- live life in the moment with a great awareness of their surroundings
- tend to believe in themselves and have a strong sense of self-worth
- are interdependent and independent and know when to be which
- easily adapt to inconvenience
- are amazingly resourceful
- are not indifferent about important issues
- have definite reasons to go on in life
- know how to weather difficult times, and are able to envision themselves being triumphant
- feel the connection to others and are appreciative of this

Of course there are many other qualities that define a survivor and any time spent with one will reveal this. They are holding the essentials for an imposing creative mind; some without ever knowing. They just live this way. I am not one of them. I had to learn how to be an imposing force. I possessed the raw materials, and at one point in my life, threw them together in a haphazard attempt to live through cancer and disseminating shingles. Somehow it came together for me, and I escaped the indescribable.

I had the basics that one would need, but I was in no way a skilled survivor. I think I may have also had a little luck on my side as well. A chance bout with shingles seemed to have stimulated my immune system into an acute, massive, immune response. I know this helped me, but I believe above all else that my spirit guided my creative mind into action and directed the inherent mind.

An unlikely tool was discovered when I sought escape from an uninspiring situation in the past. I was offered—by my mind—something that as children we use often to create from boredom. It was imagination. I found it to be a very effective means of coping with an undesirable predicament. It takes the mind to a safe place. It's something I wouldn't have thought could be so helpful. I had always held the opinion that imagination was idle. I didn't see its place in this situation until I needed it. With imagination, I could create; I could set a tone in my mind. This can support thoughts of self-reliance.

I won't have to rely so much on chance or luck anymore, because I see now what saved me—and how. I'll take all of these fine attributes and make them mine.

Disease is a struggle of attrition. The strength of your will to live will be tested beyond any comprehension you might have had before. Disease will attempt to wear down, first your body, then your emotions, and lastly, it will trespass into the sacred dwelling where your spirit exists. You stand against this happening. Be imposing, be creative and resilient. Use everything you have to defy it. All these are essentials to living through adversity.

INHERIT THE MYSTERY

Life without God is uninspiring.

There exists a mystery beyond the grips of humanity, but not beyond its benefitting from it. So many throughout time have tried to make it their own, to do unnatural things to its truth, but it has been an effort in vain. That's because it's something which cannot be possessed. We can only capture our idea of what this mystery is. But when we do this, when we try to hold it in place, we look at the mystery through perception; we are only looking at what once was. With that perception begins its distortion. We interpret according to our limited understanding, and interpretation of something that lives *only* in the now—will always be flawed; because it is always changing. So, we end up knowing only its shadow—never what casts it; we are able to see its wake, but not what makes it. To really know the mystery is to live in the here and now; that's where it will always be.

To inherit this mystery we must be in tune with the higher laws of humanity; our spirit must be vital, and we must be living with the best in us at work. The individual will be hard-pressed to come to a state of mind where these divine qualities of humanity are with him or her unless the individual is willing to be selfless. To be selfless is to feel deeply for others, to love without conditions, without expecting in return. This is a love born of creativity and appreciation for life—not just your own but others as well.

Set aside all thoughts of possession for the moment. Let this go. Now think of the pain and sorrow of loss that a neighbor or a stranger might be experiencing at this moment. Don't turn away from this thought but embrace the feeling. Know this is happening somewhere to someone. This is more than you, but it should affect you when you are sensitive, when you have compassion. If you should have in your heart a strong desire to lessen this suffering, then you have this mystery within you; there is immeasurable beauty in you. You are with God.

To be caught within this mystery, requires an understanding of the higher laws. To see life as it is, without judgment, without condemnation, is the beginning of truth. Temperance—of the emotions that wither our spirit and can bring us disease—is part of this new vision.

We have the ability to influence the world rather than the world having influence over us. To be imposing requires confidence. When the individual creates a new way forward through original actions, through self-reliance, through intelligence of a different kind, he or she brings about like responses from others. That is how things change.

Our natural inclination is to try and tame this mystery, this healing energy that performs miracles. We attempt to do this because we want certainty and stability. We want to feel as if we are in control of what happens to us. In a way we are; in other ways, we are not. There are realities and then there are illusions. Our control comes from within; this is a reality. The illusion of control comes from without. You cannot control your environment, but you can control how you respond to it. This depends on whether or not you are assertive or you are reactionary. Most everything is a state of mind.

Control is not always a sign of strength; sometimes it is the opposite. We try to control our surroundings because we lack confidence within ourselves. We try to control out of fear. True strength comes when we expose ourselves to life, without fear or façade, but instead purely and genuinely. We are assured by what is within; that is all we need; nothing else is necessary.

The mystery in life is a force of living truth. It is a movement that never detracts. It can only do so as it flows through the individual. There it can be hindered and drastically depleted. This happens when we are not living with the best in us at work. The healing energy cannot flow freely through the body when it is tense, hesitant, worried, doubtful, and fearful; when it is with anger, hate, jealousy, or portraying any of the emotions that wither. This healing energy is the bearer of life itself. Without its benefits, the body perishes. This is real.

You will not find the momentum of the mystery in habit or routine, fear or hesitation. It cannot be found in any establishment or institution—no matter how traditional. It exists in the living, within the present moment, but nowhere can it be found in the past or the future—only there can be found traces of what was or what might be; but this is not truth.

To know the great healing force of God is to stand before it innocent and wondrous as a child, yet with the intelligence of a fully mature and balanced mind and spirit, living with the higher laws. This innocence I refer to is not one that we are familiar with. Innocence that follows you through life is when you know humankind through and through, yet you are master over that knowledge; you are unaffected by this knowledge. Innocence that remains with us is when we are aware of all that surrounds us, yet we are steady, we are sure, we rise above temptation. Pure innocence is what will always grace us even while every aspect of life moves through our minds, and still we remain naturally sanctified. The innocence that is eternal stays with us beyond childhood, in spite of any age barrier. It is what keeps us young at heart. We will never lose this if we live with the best in us facing the world.

There really is no distance between you and this great mystery we know as God. It is and always will be within you. There is no need to search for the answer; it is so close that it shadows the question. Reach within yourself to inherit the mystery; reach out to share the strength and glory of that discovery. Be in the moment and you will be with God; the healing energy will flow through you without restraint. Miracles are most attainable in this way.

THE BEST IN US

Change yourself and you change the world.

Where are you now? You who one morning brought in to me your own gathering of wild flowers from well outside my pale, barren room; who, with just one gesture, freed me from the depths of the sameness of each passing day. And the only fare you asked was a kiss in return, as you leaned over to touch my lips with yours, ever softly. I was no more than seventeen then, but I certainly sensed the attraction you showed me.

Where've you gone now that I'm a man and need more than ever your sweet offering? I was young and at war when you came into my life, into my room—smiling so lively. To see you in this way made me feel as if the day had just sprung into existence. The very moment our mouths met, all of the pain had left me.

What you gave to me was rare, although, in my eyes, more than appropriate. You impressed me by showing me consideration, but most of all, in you I saw a living God.

I will always remember you, even though this happened to me so many years ago. It was the one thing which set you apart from the other nurses, whose silhouettes are all that is left of their presence in my memory. But if I saw you again, I would know you right away. Every curve of your face, the tint of your eyes, your faint scent of a woman, I would know, because you showed me the best in you, the way you reached out beyond your profession with such a special compassion. You were mindful when I was alone and unsure of my fate and your deed was more than enough to thoroughly distract me.

But did you know that because of this, I would remember you forever? Did you realize then that one gesture could be so potent in my thoughts—that I would be writing about you some decades later?

I thought about that nurse, not as much then as I did when I remembered what little things made the difference in my life. How far-reaching one extraordinary act of compassion can be in a world preoccupied with itself and its own concerns. It's easy to see why we're so unfamiliar with whom we really are and what our purpose for being here just might be, with everything pulling us in so many different directions; though I will say that there are times like these that bring us much closer to really living.

There is a need to reach out to one another. Human contact is so important in this way. The impact of these simple gestures can be remarkable. Their effects echo throughout the life of the giver *and* the receiver.

I was rushed to the emergency room by my mother during an acute attack of radiation enteritis. I was in my late twenties at the time. There was a possibility that I was obstructed as well; this made things very serious. Wide-eyed with concern, I couldn't stay still on the cart they placed me on; the pain was too much to be cool about it. I tried to deep-self-massage my abdomen, to relieve the restricted area; sometimes this helped me. In doing so, the pain becomes much more intense, but to me it's well worth it just to be unobstructed.

My mother remained in the waiting area. Even though she was tired and had to work the next day—she stayed. It was very early in the morning and I had waited quite a while because I didn't speak up; no one knew just how uncomfortable I had been.

Finally a woman approached me. At first I thought it was my nurse, but then she introduced herself as my doctor for the night. She was vaguely familiar, but I knew so many people in the hospital that I couldn't quite place her. She leaned over and whispered that she knew me, that I would be all right, and that she would see to it personally.

"Don't you know me?" She said. I told her that she looked familiar, but I didn't recognize her. "You did something that I will never forget. You sent me a card after one of your emergency room visits several years ago, expressing your appreciation for the care that I gave you. It came at a time when I needed very much to hear that I made a difference in someone's life. I've kept it on my night table ever since. It inspires me when I get weary, and reminds me that I am serving a purpose that is felt deeply by some."

I may have been completely distracted by my circumstance, but I couldn't have felt better right then and there. I did remember her. Whenever I thought someone had gone above and beyond their duty—I noticed. I felt like I should let them know—so I did.

We may not realize it, but each one of us has so much to offer. Time and time again I've been rejuvenated by the most unassuming people. To me they can be so beautiful. We don't see this in ourselves; we don't realize that our words can move mountains if they are felt as genuine, if they are sensed to be from the heart. I could always tell the difference. I knew immediately when someone's thoughts and words were not their own, but borrowed from the multitudes. And this left me at times—uninspired and still waiting for the real thing.

But when a nurse, another patient, or a doctor looked into my eyes and seemed to struggle with their emotions as they spoke to me, it was like they were giving to me a piece of themselves. It did more for me than they could ever imagine. I felt their truth come to the surface of that moment, and this made me feel alive and a special bond with them.

What would happen if we loved each other and ourselves the way we say we should love God? I'm sure that we try the best we can, taking into consideration the world around us and the way it affects our perception of things. While our intentions are admirable, they are not nearly enough to reap the benefits of the higher laws we so desperately need to remain with, in order to realize robust health. When you love yourself—and I don't mean with vanity—you love the mystery, the healing force, the creativeness within you that needs your guidance and confident embrace. When you can love yourself in this way, you are in a better place to reach out to others and love them as well.

We must first love ourselves, look beyond our faults and our superficial appearance; we must strip every layer of bad memory, negative emotion, and false projection of our-self, to get to the core of who we really are. These heavy layers are burdensome. They will not reveal what is within us all—only conceal our natural beauty. When we are bare of all that is not our true selves, we are our strongest, and then with God. It was this healing force within me which compelled me to find it. I never knew that it was in me. I had always thought that it was somewhere else. It is this notion of God within us all, which persuades us to search for it. All along, it has always been right here with me. I just wasn't aware.

This vital truth stirs within our spirit; this is the healing force tugging at your attention, just waiting to unleash its beauty, its creativity, its strength.

The conflict that produces strife within us is that undercurrent of truth compelling us to search for things that are real and genuine; knowing, sensing, in the end, that very search will lead us home, right back to our spirit.

When we feel compassion toward another in need, when we live with the virtues, when we withstand emotions that wither, we live with the best in us—we live with God.

God is the greatest mystery, the healing force, life's energy; exactly what you never understood about yourself but couldn't wait to find out. God is the restless force within you that you did not understand or were afraid to let free. God is the wild and untamed passion that society tries to subdue in very subtle ways so that you do not notice or rebel against these ways. Society's force subtly distracts us all so that it will not awaken this sleeping giant. It seeks attention from the individual in the form of conformity and security in tradition in all its ways. It resists change as much as it can, so therefore lives—mostly without truth.

We say that we want change but it is only the idea of change that many seek; because, to really change would be too uncomfortable and require an upheaval of habit, of routine. But you will not find the totality of God while in immersed in habit—only impressions of it. You will not see the truth of the moment if you are wedged in routine. You will be too rigid—not supple in mind.

God is in the living moment, that is, a vital force that is very much alive—within us all. Everything shows me this; nothing has shown me otherwise. The presence of God is evident when the best in us is revealed through right thinking leading to right actions. God is a living movement of vitality and grace. God is there for us in our most desperate situations. God can be found in the acts of compassion, in the touch of healing hands, an attentive listener, a thoughtful gesture, comforting words, in the feat of forgiveness, a tender, gentle kiss, even an endearing smile, and too, in an inconvenient sacrifice. The life force is strong in those who know themselves well enough to stand alone if need be, holding to their convictions, if those convictions are from the core of themselves.

This idea of God should be in every breath I take and in every creative thought that leads to a just action. It reawakens the imagination that once was a part of me. Most of all, it is a promise of life that is everlasting and not at all ephemeral. It has been with us since the beginning. Its presence has cast many shadows among past and present cultures and religions. It's given us a sense of what is, but its true essence has more often eluded us.

Many of us have become fond of the idea of God and not what is real. God is not at all a convenience, a part of a schedule, or within the foundation of an institution. God is the force of life that comes through you when your spirit welcomes it.

There can be a great distance between the idea of something and the reality of it. One cannot know the sway of the human spirit and its reign over the body without feeling God deeply and passionately; it is one in the same. Living with truth, that is, living in the moment, and not turning away from need, is the beginning of knowing the real, and revealing the healing potential of the greatest mystery, that is God. That need can be toward others or guided inwardly, spiritually, which is the attention given to the internal relating entities responsible for vibrant health.

I realize now that I must put forth the best in me in order to align myself with the healing force; I must know who I am by the way that I relate to others and the way I relate with myself. My true existence is in the reflection of these very relations.

I think we all crave something real in our lives. That is what's missing from many of our lives. Maybe there are those who need us in a way that only we are capable of offering them. I know how we long to be close to each other, but aren't quite sure just how to do so. I believe we desire to be relied upon and also to rely on others, and yet we remain so distant from this truth—so distant from each other.

It's hard for us to admit this because there's so much vulnerability exposed; so most of us keep this craving to ourselves. But keeping this to ourselves will not change things; it will only suffocate the best qualities that should define us. How can we ever know God if we allow this to happen?

Let everything go that is not really who you are and expose the best in you to the world. Let the world see God through you. Trust that this is what will work. It has worked for me.

TRUST

I t took a long time for me to believe in myself and know exactly how to trust in what nature provides us to overcome disease. In order to have the kind of confidence that will carry you through the adversity I experienced, you must find out what it is about you that should be trusted in these uncertain times; an endeavor that can be very revealing.

I had no one in my life who had gone through something similar to what was happening to me. I was supported, but no one self-assured me. We were all in the dark with what was next to come. No one could see around life's corner; there were many sharp turns and unexpected detours along the way.

There will be times in your life when you will have to be the path-finder. You will be in a situation where you will find yourself treading on unfamiliar ground; seize that moment. It may be your path of self-discovery.

We think that we have boundaries, until we break them or see someone else live through the unthinkable. Then we begin to trust more in ourselves and in what is possible. Sometimes there is nothing to go by and *you* are the one who must reach within and show the way for yourself and possibly for others.

The limitations of your mind must be stretched in order to persevere. To do this, you must be willing to rely on yourself.

Every day people are living through cancer; they are finding a way to live. Some survive to the astonishment of their doctors, even after they were given a death sentence.

There is something special that doctors do not have at their disposal when treating disease. It is something that you cannot lend to someone in these situations, and yet it makes all the difference in the world. No one can give to you what you—and only you—can give to yourself. This ability lies within the mind and spirit of the individual. Medicine will never be able to give to the patient the will to live—to defy. It cannot tend to the human spirit as it can tend to the human body. That is something only the individual is capable of doing. That is where the true strength of the individual exists.

When we trust in something wholeheartedly, it is usually if there's something about that belief which makes us certain beyond any doubt. But do we have the confidence to believe in ourselves like we do in the knowledge that the sky we look toward is blue or the grass we tread barefoot on is green? This we can see for ourselves, so we are convinced. How can we believe in the type of inner strength that eludes the five senses, in the same way—with the same conviction? Not everything real can be corroborated by these physical receptors. But like the creative/inherent mind and the human spirit—both intangible, yet very much a factor of our survival, there is the sixth sense that can override all of the other senses. Call it our gut feelings, instinct or intuition, but it is real and does provide us with a keen sense of our surroundings—both within and without; in the physical world and what is unseen.

I have developed trust in my sixth sense. Through the years it has served me well. I've made life changing decisions based on my intuition and have come out all right because of it. I now have that confidence in this ability. I consider it just as important—if not, than more—as I do my other five senses. I use everything that is at my disposal because I believe that life made each one of us self-reliant when it comes to surviving. Life equips us with whatever is necessary to overcome; we just have to know what it is that defends us. This takes awareness.

When living with so many distractions in life and so much stress, it's not so easy to follow your natural abilities. They can be dulled by society. Your natural responses to life are corrupted by too muddled an environment. You must be clear of these outward stimuli. You have to be inwardly convinced of where you are headed. You must be guided by one undistracted mind. You must have faith in your ability to heal yourself with that absolute deep, rich, confidence; nothing short of this will do when it comes to trusting yourself. To believe this, you must know yourself intimately; you must be familiar with every aspect of your existence. You must be ever aware of the inner nuances of your body, mind, and of course, your spirit within.

There was a time when all that I considered relevant to survival remained outside of me. An external reliance kept me reactive and vulnerable against the whim of circumstance. But then what little confidence I had—my physical strength—eroded right in front of me. This left me naked in life. I was stripped of the strengths I had nurtured through my adolescence. When the time came that I would need an inconceivable strength, one absolutely necessary to go through such a catastrophic condition as cancer, trust in myself was really put to the test. Whatever I relied upon had to be real and sustainable, as life was thrown at me.

Before being diagnosed with cancer, I responded to life with predictability. I let life happen to me. I didn't know there was another attitude to have that was better for me. I didn't see that I must be as unpredictable as life itself. I must be a reflection of nature—not an opposing or reactive force, but one that flows with life. I must be forever creating, just as life does. I must never fall into complacency or indifference. I must be more than habit, routine, and following ritual—the very things that make the mind and spirit stagnant and stale.

This would take a greater confidence of knowing my strengths and trusting God within me. But I didn't understand that life shows no mercy for those passing tentatively through nature's domain. I didn't understand that there were higher laws beyond the distractions. Self-doubt contradicts this kind of intelligence. This intelligence I refer to

can only be realized when living in the moment with an acute awareness to the present. It is a healing force with enormous potential for
much, if not, all of human kind's ills. The individual has the responsibility to find a way to understand this, simply because the path to its
discovery—lies inward.

To know that so many have lived through cancer is comforting
and inspiring. It lets us know that it can be done. But it must be said
that in order for the many to support the one, the one needs to believe
in oneself to have any real chance of survival. To do this, you must
know yourself enough to be confident in your ability. The way through
has been shown by survivors, people just like anybody else. They are
no different and possess no special gift. There is a common denominator in most of the survivors of cancer. Each has shown a tenacious
determination to live. They never think of giving in—no matter what.
They are impervious to outside suggestions and fears, if these are
defeating in any way. Such people know exactly what attitude should
be cultivated from within. Their similar way of looking at their
predicament is no coincidence. Through their stories, be reassured by
the fact that anything is possible and miracles are more common than
once thought. Learn from them their methods of coping and dealing
with adversity, and awaken the same qualities within yourself, to do the
same thing, which is, ultimately, to fight for your life.

There should be no doubt in your mind—no hesitation. Impose
your will through every turn of events. Never let fear grab hold of
your mind. Live with this certainty at all times. Know who you are;
know what you can do. Above all, do not be afraid. Fear can be a
hindrance when it hangs around too long and overstays its welcome.

Be aware that there will come a point when the mind only gets in
the way. This may happen in the darkest hours. Let go of this worry;
release it. Then relax yourself. Let the great intelligence that is within
you do what it does best. Stay in the company of your disease. Be with
it; let it know that you are watching it and that it will not take you.

Stare it down in your mind. Let it know that it has no place in your body. Be sure of yourself. Life will listen to you; your body will surge and obey your wishes because it will sense your confidence and determination. It needs this very direction. All of this matters. This is the way to purge disease—by being imposing. Remember what disease is trying to do; it is trying to take your life! Do something about it! Defy it!

Reflect inner poise, in the midst of uncertainty. The inherent mind will follow the creative mind and your will, because it is subordinate to those who are sure of what they want, in those whose spirituality is strong.

True confidence comes from being intimately aware of what is taking place within you from moment to moment. It comes from trusting yourself in a way that one must, in order to live through the hardest of times. It is within your reach, so reach for it!

NEVER LET
WORDS KILL YOU

I remember allowing words to cloud my ability to see past them—to the truth of my fears; grave words like death, and the different types of cancers, paralyzed me, when I heard of them. My creative mind gave way to these anxieties. I lent strength to these words by fearing them, by not understanding. This compromised the way I handled life then.

In order for something to take hold of our attention and distract us from the essence of life, we must first give it power to do so. While the mystery of God and its healing energy remains unaffected throughout time, we humans have many affectations of influence all around us. Our spirit is bombarded by distractions from our true priorities of survival. We do not have the luxury to indulge these destructive thoughts or passive suggestions by others. We may think that we do, but we don't; there are always consequences for deviations from focusing.

Cancer has earned a certain respect in our minds, mainly because we've seen and heard of its wrath since our youth. As children we look on as this bad thing ravages and destroys families and lives around us. We see that adults are afraid and when they speak of it, they do so in whispers, as if not to awaken the sleeping giant or stir an inner superstition. Then we think that if they are fearful, then it must be serious. So we learn this fear early on in our childhood, either directly or indirectly. The anxiety is greater if you feel deeply or realize your own mortality early on, like me. I was bothered by the ability that cancer possessed, to bring us to our knees—as a society.

As children, we haven't the emotional tools to understand this intruding force, nor can we see it or lay our hands on it to know that is dangerous, as we could, a hot stove or lit candle. It is this unknown that seeps into our inherent mind. This fear, like a weed, begins to sprout and grow roots where our productive garden should be. Each time we hear of this 'cancer' and its effects, we feed the fear and our beautiful garden slowly withers, as we hand over more power to this intruder, because we think that we have no control over it. What frightens us the most is the belief that we are more or less powerless against it. This concession of confidence is what eventually suffocates our life force.

As I mentioned earlier, I was quite young when I first became aware of cancer. My grandfather caused a scare in the family when it was thought that he might have cancer. I remember vividly, as we were an extremely close Italian family, the events surrounding his hospital stay. Many of us gathered for support and, of course, to eat as well, but what stands out the most was my grandmother's anguish over the possibility of losing my grandpa. I didn't understand. Growing up, we fourteen grandchildren have always known our grandfather to be strong—very strong. He was a stout, agile, man, with gorilla-like hands that could wrestle down a horse if need be. I'm sure that he has, from what we've been told about his early years in the cavalry. There were many fascinating stories passed down on his behalf. Most were a bit dramatic, but we all could see through the embellishments to the truth of his deeds.

In a way, I could see to the truth of cancer through my mother's attempt to reassure us that everything would be alright. Children are intuitive and sensitive to nuances of conversation. I suppose that we all forget how perceptive we were when we were young; perhaps even more so, than as we age.

Everyone who knew my grandfather or knew of him solidified our belief that he was a formidable man. So why was my grandmother so concerned? What was it about this thing called cancer that everyone trembled at the thought of; that might even bring down my legendary grandfather? This is how cancer, for me, became something of an entity of its own, without a conscience, acting almost independently of society, and therefore, beyond its control—its understanding. Is that not the perception we have towards it? Can't that fear get out of hand?

Over the years, this fear and misunderstanding was fueled by the many stories of those who had succumbed to it. I had always been aware of my childhood best friend's mother, who died from cancer just after he was born. I always wondered about that. I felt bad for him, that he never knew his real mom. I didn't think that it was fair. Why would cancer take someone's mother away? This scared me. I thought about my mom. I thought about losing her too.

In time, I began to be conditioned by the rumors which eventually swallowed the inner confidence of the impressionable boy that I had been. Fear imposed itself on my life. It was not spit out like poison, nor was it spent appropriately, because I was not mature enough to reason it away, or even confront it, as we must do in life if we're to neutralize its effect.

I carried this fear with me. I kept it close by, deep within my thoughts. But I did not hold it—it held me. And a mind that is fearful—is doubtful, worried, and hesitant. Eventually, the body will absorb these feelings directly, into every living cell.

It is a scientific fact that on an ongoing basis our bodies ward off cancer as it develops.

Our immune system, when properly functioning with the help of a balanced mind and staunch will, is able to arrest any forward progression of a cancer cell as it attempts to further invade surrounding areas of the body. The immune system has been performing this function since the beginning of mankind. It is very familiar with cancer and remembers how to combat it.

Unfortunately, there are influences in life, many dynamics, which get in the way of an otherwise properly operating system of checks and balances within the body. As the gears of society's machine grind and churn in unpredictable, erratic ways, its clumsy implementation can have far-reaching effects on our health. A whole revolution of the mind as well as a side step away from the rat race of society is needed, for a complete and right recuperation.

This is a vast transformation of perception. This level of change is most often resisted and sometimes feared by the inherent mind. It is the unknown which causes us to hesitate and doubt our abilities. But we deserve so much more than this. We settle for so much less than what is possible.

Even the unacceptable procedures of today, such as radiation and chemotherapy, can be more comfortable to some than to face the uncertainty of a less traveled road. I understand this, but I must tell you that life is not like that at all. It pushes forward relentlessly, imposing itself upon us with no malice or mercy. It is a force. If we are willing, this force will take us through everything and anything with the intelligence of God.

Fear of death can be consuming and counterproductive. Chronic, underlying fear, worry or anxiety takes away from living and weakens our resolve. It steals valuable time from us.

Instead, we should spend our fear wisely. We should use fear for what it was intended to do, and that is to instigate an appropriate action for the immediate threat. If there is no threat, then, see through the fear, to the truth of why it is there. Follow the problem to the end, and maybe when you see the real reason that we fear, that exposure will bring a better understanding of yourself. In that understanding, you may once and for all free yourself. But when you worry about the past catching up, or you become overly concerned about the future, that's when fear and doubt will again trespass where it doesn't belong. When you live in the moment and create from the enormous energy of the present, then you will not be concerned about yesterday or tomorrow, because you will be caught up in the immense appreciation of life that is here and now.

I realize that we can never be fearless all the time, but we can spend fear when it arises. Use it to instigate a creative action which empowers instead of immobilizes. Patients with limited, very, curable cancers have died. Conversely, there are patients with terminal cancers who have survived in spite of the odds. What this tells me is that there is much more going on than we are aware of. It tells me that nothing is predictable. It tells me that we all have unseen, unnoticed strengths that need our attention.

We have more than a fighting chance of overcoming cancer of any kind and at any stage, if we have confidence in place of fear. These intangible strengths are very much necessary when it comes to defeating a tangible disease such as cancer.

Cancer comes to us and we eradicate it. We are victorious over this disease. Know this. Believe this. Have this confidence in yourself. You will persevere in the end, if you know that you will; if you believe this. Fear can either paralyze you if you allow it, or it can give to you— energy to fight. Use the inspiration of fear to defy. Never defeat yourself by letting words breach your creative mind and penetrate through to your inherent mind. Use wisely, deliberately, your strong spirit to prevent this.

A.M.I.R.

Acute Massive Immune Response

W e're all aware of instances when miraculous recoveries from cancer have been achieved, despite the most discouraging circumstances. They are often reluctantly documented—with an unstructured explanation, awkwardly interpreted with mystical undertones and an ambiguous haze surrounding them. Still, the evidence is there; undeniable at that.

These extraordinary stories are taking place the world over; case histories of hopeless terminal patients sent home to die, who instead lived through their death sentence, to astonish the medical establishment. Of course anyone can dismiss what cannot be seen, as a fluke, but it becomes more difficult to dismiss it again and again, as if fact wasn't a requisite to truth. Something is happening in these situations, something well worth our investigation, falling far beyond the understanding of traditional medicine.

What happened to me in that isolation room when I was so close to dying, could, under no circumstances, be considered suspect. Everything had taken place within the hospital, under the watchful eyes of the professionals around me, fully documented by nurses, doctors, and yes, even researchers. There were no external variables to explain this away so easily.

I was admitted with shingles and a cluster of malignant lymph nodes beneath my left underarm, and discharged almost four weeks later, with the shingles retreating and my underarm completely clear of the cancerous mass. Something exceptionally potent happened in that room; something actual. I don't have to see to believe it; there need not be a smoking gun. I've learned there are other ways to know truth, other senses we can rely on besides our basic five. When you collect circumstantial evidence of the presence of something and all that evidence points to something occurring, then it becomes no leap of faith to know with some degree of certainty what has taken place.

When seemingly incredible recoveries occur in life, many will point to whatever it was at the time that they had tried, in a desperate measure to survive, but therein lies the distraction from an underlying truth which seems to be overlooked in all the excitement. They will say that it was by the grace of God, and that may be somewhat and indirectly true, but there is much more at work here, much more within our grasp, then a miracle of mercy.

I've heard endless theories and accounts of why this happens to some and not others, ranging anywhere from the ingestion of rare bark from a tree in the Amazons to a seed from the pit of a common fruit taken in large quantities. There is great confusion with this way of thinking—a great distraction from what is really happening. Yes, I do believe that many of these teas, tonics and concoctions are good for the body in some way, and one might benefit from following these measures with a long-term objective. But in no way am I convinced that diet change or taking in any potion from the earth, as of yet, will suddenly cure cancer.

A clear distinction must be made between crisis and prevention, when considering alternatives to more conventional therapies. Now, is it possible that any one of these natural remedies might very well help to stimulate the internal systems into action? Of course, anything is possible; to what extent I cannot say. I would place more value— much more value—on what I am about to suggest is at the heart of this so called, "instantaneous cure" of cancer.

There is only one logical and reasonable explanation for a sudden recovery from cancer, after therapies have been exhausted or one has embarked on a self-healing endeavor. I believe strongly that this is the work of the internal systems kicking into overdrive, in what I term the "live or die syndrome." It is not unlike the familiar, "fight or flight syndrome," of which lends us, albeit temporarily, a super-human strength. Consider this: What if, like the fight or flight syndrome, we also have at our ready a comparable phenomenon implemented internally. In lieu of spontaneous remission, the name given for the sudden, unexplained disappearance of cancer, I suggest that what has actually taken place here might be considered an "acute, massive, immune response." There is nothing spontaneous about this occurrence at all. In fact it is a clear indication of the inner systems working in coordination to overcome a threat against the human organism. I have the opinion that our immune system does indeed have an overdrive. I believe what happens during a so-called do or die scenario is nothing short of amazing, in that what we're really witnessing is a fight or flight syndrome on a physiological level.

It's very probable that, as I've discussed earlier in the book, the inherent mind senses trouble within the body, through some realm of intuition we have yet to master, and delivers messages via the nervous system, which in turn fires up the endocrine system. This action progresses to eventually stimulate the immune system into action. It is a concerted effort of a sequence of actions based on specific relations within the body, when the relating entities come together to wage an uprising against this threat to life. It is an all-out effort given, a second wind, that kicks in near the end, or possibly even sooner, depending on how reactive the internal systems are in their response. The immune system responds by churning out more B-cells, T-cells, and macrophages, which utilize the blood stream to blast the cancerous tissues with a surge of powerful anticancer fighters.

One of the down sides to conventional therapies is the fact that these treatments we use today to treat cancer, though helpful to a degree, tend to decrease the body's ability to mount a legitimate immune response that might send someone into an A.M.I.R. The common and accepted use of conventional therapies, e.g. radiation and chemotherapy, can unfortunately be a double-edged sword and might even ultimately prevent this so called 'last stand' from ever taking place.

A more subtle version of this acute, massive, immune response has been witnessed in the elderly by caregivers in nursing homes where the patient is closely monitored. Many times you will hear someone say that the patient never looked better right before their passing. They had gained an unusual amount of vitality for the condition they were in, enough to be noticed. It's an interesting occurrence. Unfortunately, in this situation the body is very old and the internal system's effort to mount a surge may be too much for the body to handle. However, in a body and mind still vital, this acute, massive, immune response can be just what we need to overcome imminent death.

Without question, the overriding common denominator which exists within patients that have defied the odds is that they all have an absolute and undeniable will to live. They will not relent. It is one time in life when being stubborn really is a good thing.

This 'will to live' far surpasses the instinct to survive, in the same way the instinctual immune system gives way to the adaptive immune system. As mammals, we have the instinct to survive as our base defense, but we have more—much more to draw from, than any other species. We have developed an adaptable intelligence and a thought-filled appreciation for life. We think, reflect, and predict. Above all, we question. This makes us responsible. We know that we must do things to stay alive, and can make choices on whether we do them or not.

We realize the consequences of death and know the stakes are very high in this game of survival. We have the ability to choose our emotions and thoughts. Beyond our basic feelings, which are instinctual and more involuntary, we have the virtuous ones. To live with virtue guiding you requires higher thought.

We have what other life forms are without—spirituality. The qualities of the human spirit are distinct to our race and set us apart from all other living things. We possess traits which make us tenacious and determined in the face of adversity. We possess attitudes of independence that follow us through generations and centuries. We demand to have a say in our lives—as we should—even regarding the manner in which we die. When defending one's life, it is no time to be meek or passive. The higher laws insist that we impose our will against death; they require that we fight to the very last breath if we have to.

Science has cracked opened the door to a once obscure concept, and has introduced the findings under the heading of Psychoneuroimmunology, or PNI, an impressive word for the relating entities working in balance. PNI attempts to scientifically identify the relationship between the central nervous system and the immune system. Science is discovering that the central nervous system is delivering messages in an ongoing basis directly to the immune system by way of tiny electrical impulses. It is a remarkable thing to know, but essential to live.

Furthermore, science seeks to decipher the ever changing states of mind which affect the internal systems. We see now that there is an actual connection in the way neurotransmitters and receptors link the central nervous system directly to the endocrine system and the immune system. More extraordinary is the remembrance of that interplay. This, evidently, is noted when observing the adaptive immune system, in the building up of specific antibodies from battles already waged against both antigens and pathogens. Science may define this interaction between the internal systems with an analytical approach, and may even develop a comprehensive format ready for the conveyor belt-type therapy, which we are all so used to by now; but the one thing it will never be able to do is provide someone with the elusive human spirit, the necessary component for an A.M.I.R. to take place.

Science will marvel at the ability of the body to regenerate itself, but it can never cross the threshold into the spiritual realm. It must watch technically, from a distance. But the patient must have a robust spirit. The patient must feel a strong connection to the life force, which is, spirituality.

So clearly, this leaves us responsible for our own lives. We must realize that to rely solely on science or the medical profession will not always be enough to rid us of a disease such as cancer.

In our hearts and minds we must prepare for adversity. You would not enter into war without a shield, armor, a weapon, or a clear strategy. This is no way to engage cancer, as well.

So how does one prepare for this adversity? You know, it is in our nature to search here and there for a better way. We tend to think that it's never right in front of us. *"How could it be?"* We think. We feel that it has got to be somewhere where we must "find" the secret to health. Well, in a way, yes, it is somewhere where you must find it. It is within you. Not all searches are meant to be outward.

Survivors are stumbling through cancer as I did. I was very fortunate in that the conditions were right for me to experience an acute, massive, immune response, and for this I lived through cancer to talk about it and share my blessing. Those who do make it through tend not to look back to make sense of their survival. That means that many others will end up stumbling through as well, and therefore might not make it through.

I felt a sense of responsibility to find out what had happened to me, and also, if I could possibly prevent it from happening again in the future. I realized that what I learned was universal, and could help so many others as well. That responsibility was accepted, and this is the action I have taken in response.

There is a clear way through. We don't need to stumble through disease any longer. In order to do this we must trace the steps of the survivors such as me. We are the *go to* people, and thus hold some of the most important lessons to unraveling the mystery of surviving through cancer—physically, emotionally and spiritually.

So now that we've seen how the human spirit prevails over all other aspects, we have to look into the many ways the human spirit relates to the mind and body. We must also better define the qualities of the human spirit and observe what it is that makes it so imposing. With such a powerful tool at our ready, it is important to familiarize oneself in this way. I feel that it is vital that each one of us sense spirituality within us.

It doesn't have to be religious in nature. It can be a connection to others or a connection to life. Let this spirituality be your religion. Above all else, do not leave your spirit empty. That would be a waste of the greatest endowment we've been given in life.

In conclusion, I want to talk about something I touched on earlier. It is about a phrase that we hear often while competing in sports. It's widely accepted that when we see a player perform flawlessly and gracefully, with no hint of hesitance in his movements, we refer to this condition as being "in the zone." Being a competitor myself, I have felt this state of mind. Being in the zone is attaining a focus without any internal or external distractions hindering the flow of confidence throughout the body and mind. There is no conflict or mixed messages between the creative/inherent mind; both are relating in perfect harmony.

The correlation can be made then that in any situation where the body/mind is called upon to perform at its best, whether it be in competition or in the act of surviving cancer, ideally, one should do what is necessary to find this state of mind which puts one directly "in the zone." What exactly constitutes being in the zone? In order to be in the zone, when it comes to dealing with illness, the mind must be light and lean; the layers of fear and doubt stripped away from the inner workings of the mind. There must be an inner focus that lends itself to the inherent mind without the creative mind getting in the way. The human spirit shifts from the creative mind to guiding the inherent mind to do what the inherent mind does best, and that is survive. In this case, the attention is focused within, all the way down to a molecular level, where the cells are very receptive to direction. They are listening to the direction of the creative/inherent mind. They can sense this confidence of being in the zone, and will respond like disciplined soldiers. In sports, physical and emotional tension can prevent this from happening; in illness, emotional tension gets in the way of being in the zone. The negative emotions become the walls that prevent the healing force from flowing throughout the body, smoothly and unencumbered. That is why it is so important to relax and trust that inner intelligence to do the right thing. This confidence will be felt, right down to every living cell in the body.

Could this "in the zone" state of mind be one of the conditions needed to produce an A.M.I.R., and by extension—tap into the healing force of life? I believe very much that these positive actions can only strengthen one's chances for a full recovery from such life-threatening diseases such as cancer.

The inherent mind has all the intelligence of the universe locked within it. Guide it with your spirit. Impose your will through the influence of the creative mind. Then trust it, and let it do what it was meant to do, which is to keep you alive. The receptors are there, joining your mind to the immune system, ready and waiting for your command.

THE HUMAN SPIRIT

Anything is possible…
anything—when the spirit guides you.

The human spirit unites with the creative mind and takes the "will to survive" to new heights. The will to survive is instinctual, as is the inherent mind; but the human spirit, along with the creative mind, is the breakaway evolution of this basic intelligence and fundamental urge to live. The will to survive and the inherent mind is governed by the laws of nature and its intelligence is reactive to its environment in a most primordial way, while the human spirit and the creative mind draw from the higher laws, of which God and nature merge to become wisdom and virtuous. This form of intelligence, this wisdom, which is really creative intelligence, enables the creative mind to be self-initiating, resourceful, imaginative, discerning, reflective, inspirational, contemplative, rebellious, self-motivating, and reasonable. With the human spirit guiding it, the creative mind inquires, envisions, yearns, follows dreams, anticipates, endeavors, and so much more.

Adhering to the higher laws enables us to inherit the mystery of miracles, the healing force. The human spirit follows humanity through the ages, developing as we discover; ever changing as we advance forward. The human spirit receives its rejuvenation from spirituality; things which inspire it and move it to action become its religion. This kind of religion transcends all human pursuits and notions of permanence. It is an evolving mysterious truth of infinite, magnificent proportions.

If we aren't realizing our own spirituality, then we are lending it outwardly for others to take hold of. This can make us very unstable and reliant. We must own our spirituality. Our religion must be felt from the depths of our being.

Faith in one's religion is explosively powerful. It is so vital to believe in what you feed your spirit, because it is the spirit that is dynamic and capable of realizing God. And when we realize God, we realize ourselves, and in this way we can be healed from within.

The human spirit has freedoms which separate it from all other living things. We possess this; it is ours and ours alone. No one can strip this from you when you are imposing and confident.

The human spirit is like a flame that at times glows with slow burning embers, and can also ignite into a raging inferno. Because of its very nature, it will reflect such contrast. It may seem that, on occasion, life is trying to smother this fire, but it cannot, even when hope is lost. The human spirit is resilient. It can be revived. No other creature on earth has this ability to resurrect its spirit; once it is broken, it is gone forever. But not the human spirit; it can be rejuvenated. Hope can be restored. It is best to always remember this.

I've made my place of worship the world. When I help others in my life, I feel spiritual. Reaching out to others is my religion; I do this because I see God in us. I can't be any closer to the mystery, the healing force, than I am when I am comforting, inspiring, taking away fear, or bringing joy. This is what strengthens me, and it would not be possible without my spirituality.

BY WAY OF
THE PAPILLON

Even in the absolute hour of our death,
life comes to our salvation

Centuries upon centuries have gone by without my presence; but I am here now, if only a brief flicker in the immense span of time. The impression I leave compares to a footprint left near the lands edge, where the tides in their pendulum-like ebb and flow, slowly but surely wash away any vestige of my existence. It is this way that time erodes all that is hand felt and forged. But this in no way means that I once did not live, or that those whom I loved or who loved me will not remember; nor does it suggest that I wasn't here to breathe deep the crisp, evergreen-infused, mountainous air, laugh hardily among friends and family, feel sorrow for loss of life, or appreciate the glorious radiance of the living kingdom that we know as earth.

Life and its ever-changing seasons is pressing upon me each and every moment, ready and wanting to resolve—to revolve, and I cannot halt its momentum forever. Therefore, I'm poised to transform while silently declaring, "So I have lived—so I will die." I cannot accept one notion without the other, still claiming to be living with truth; and with the courage put forth in life, I will turn toward death in that same manner…when that time comes.

The greatest unknown lies waiting for us, inviting us home from where we originally came. Although, the fear that many of us seem to have about dying is caught up in that return, through a collective perception of what death symbolizes. In that fear we've made dying a cold and unnatural experience. Our culture has isolated it from being an intimate part of life.

In our thoughts we rarely think of our ending as a peaceful one, where we set off to some abandoned meadowland bursting with legions of wildflowers delicately bowed by the nudge of summer's warm but timely gentle breeze. Off and away are the meandering specks of the papillon, dallying about among the abundant blooms, where, not so far off in the distance we discover a lone tree draped with willows ever weeping low against the backdrop of a long neglected stone fashioned wall of boundary. It is there where we nestle ourselves under this great natural canopy. Our senses heighten, as we listen to the native birds of this low-land, sounding off at one another in a beautiful dance of relations. The echoes of the living soothe like the forgotten, early embrace against a mother's tender bosom. Reassured are we then, as our breathing slows yet—stiller, until the hallowing reed fields come forth into light, beckoning, as we drift into the dark, eternal cascading night; hence, we are no more…but evermore.

Far from this interpretation have we imagined the end; our thoughts can be most unforgiving. In our fear and misunderstanding of death, along with our denial of its inevitability, we've somehow distorted this higher law into a separate occurrence.

The idea of death has been allowed to tarnish the beauty of confidence, stealing away the living time that we seem to have so little of already. Its effects seep into every crevice of our mind, suffocating the very life force essential to our survival. We watch ever subtlety, even complacently, as we shrivel from within, powerless and consumed—by our unwillingness to put death in its respective place.

If we're honest with ourselves, we'll admit that the thought of dying has had our attention many more times than it deserves, and it has caused us to desperately seek permanence in many forms.

Death, in its place of course, is as natural as birth. Should we begin to perceive it in this way, I believe that we'd have much more appreciation for life without the thought of death ever interfering; this, because we've understood that dying is a natural part of life.

In the end therefore, life, like truth, can never be owned. We may inherit its wonder, but never own its mystery. That alone should be enough for us, though it seldom is; because it's in our nature to overlook what we have in front of us. We've liberated ourselves from our instinctual minds long ago, but in that liberation we've realized our deaths are inevitable, and this haunts us throughout our lives. It has haunted humanity all throughout time—some more than others. We are fixated on it because we cannot get past the end; but we must, in order to know the eternal, in order to truly feel what it is to be free.

How do we see this? How do we bring a sustainable peace to our life as well as to our death? Is this possible? I think first we have to understand what it means to be at peace, and then come to terms with the fact that there is a time for dying, not in theory, but in reality. We do this by seeing the whole process of life, not just the side that we want or prefer to see, which is not to say that there shouldn't always be a fierce attempt for life—to the contrary.

When we see the truth of the whole, we also realize the significance of the time that we do have, and then we want even more to appreciate it without interruption. I think also, we need not turn away from death but instead alter our own perception of it, change the way we think of it, and begin to look at this natural thing without fear; not so much to welcome it, as to accept its conditions as another part of life. Optimism should follow us through death.

Fear of death is natural, healthy, and as it so happens, necessary for survival in many ways, but like everything else that can be exaggerated or dramatized, so too can our sense of it be. The impact of this dramatization can be far-reaching.

Fear is energy of the mind and it's created to be spent quickly—so spend it! Don't harbor, fight or deny it—spend it. It sets us into action. But if we mishandle fear, it becomes something else entirely. If we diffuse fear into worry or anxiety, it becomes chronic and detrimental to health. It wears away at our spirit, our nerves, and ultimately, our immune system.

Fear must be channeled in the many directions that life could use this energy. Try not to make it more than it is; it is only the means to something, not the end. It is no more than this except when it is misunderstood, at which point it becomes the focus and more important than it should be.

Fear is instinctual. It is one of our basic emotions. It was meant to stimulate the body and mind into action during emergencies. It was never meant to be chronic. It's not an emotion like joy or contentment that can remain underlying while living day to day. All the negative emotions were meant for short term use. None were ever intended for obsessive durations.

I think most of our fears come to us because we are afraid of losing our "self", which we have created in the course of life; we are worried that one day it will all end, that we will lose this awareness. The key word here is created. Our fear of losing ourselves is possibly a manifestation of the inherent mind holding on to a creation of the creative mind's lifetime work. The inherent mind sees this collection of who we are, what we've become, and wants to keep it. It tries to seek permanence in a conditional world. It is all that it knows—to survive. It doesn't live with the higher laws; this is for the creative mind. It must rely on the creative mind and the spirit to calm it.

Some worry about immortality. They wonder if they will be remembered. They wonder if they will remember. If you are near your end, find comfort in knowing that you will live on in the ones you've touched deeply in your lifetime. Your immortality will rest on the impression you've made to those loved ones you've been blessed to know and share company with. The truth of who you are will always prove evident in the end.

I feared, through my childhood years, this idea of death that I talk about; I feared for myself and my loved ones. But when I was dying, fear was nowhere to be found in my hospital room. My mind was free to wander away into the vast imagination that we know when we are young. It was no longer concerned about what was to be. I was lean in my mind. The mystery came to my bedside to comfort me; it was real. I was at peace with all that mattered; I was at peace with myself. I didn't have guilt, fear or anxiety suffocating my life force. The healing energy flowed through me unencumbered. Everything felt natural.

I'm here to tell those courageous ones who may find themselves exhausted beyond any measure, from their personal fight for life, that there's a kind of relief you may be unaware of at the moment, but will come to you when you need it. It's real and beautiful in itself, and is part of the great mystery which transcends life and death. It is an infinite glory of both worlds and unites now with the hereafter. It is meant for those who are most passionate in their pursuits and endeavors. It forgets not those who lived in the delicate realm of truth throughout life, and is a promise of everlasting peace that begins not in death but in the act of dying.

During the times when I was nearest to death, I wavered between a focus on the moment without fear, and finding comfort in the freedom from this fear. I was at times living in the moment and then escaping to replenish my spirit.

In that final hour, if your eyes are searching for God—and I believe they will be—know that it is within you and reflected in the eyes of those around you. In their eyes you will know selfless love and enormous compassion, and this will calm your spirit more than anything else. Let it. Seize this moment; it is yours. It will last you eternally.

Trust in this. In that very instant you will have peace without end, the kind of peace which thoroughly dissolves all of your worries.

There will be memories at your ready to soothe your labored breathing. Great memories will wash away the fear and send it far away and all that will be left will be visions—beautiful visions, images that we've tucked away in our thoughts for that day that it rains heavily on us. Only then, the rain will be welcome and cleansing. We could never forget the memories that ease, because deep inside we've always known that they were meant to be reserved for that special day. Something told us that the most indelible times in our lives were to be held tight in our minds until we needed them the most.

I have a memory I'd like to share with you. Each time I remembered this scene, it moved me; it still does. It helped me through when I was alone and uncertain, when there was not much to inspire me. It helped me when things began to look bleak:

There was a time when I was walking through the woods, right around dusk. I was accompanied by a close friend and his dogs. It was a brisk late November evening and the path was slowly beginning to shadow. The dogs were playful yet weary from a long day chasing game. We both were tired and without words as our heads bent low from fatigue and to see our steps in the dimness. I glanced just high enough to catch a glimpse of some flickering reflections against the sky, when I was struck by a revelation ahead of me; between the naked trees and above the laurel, way off in the distance was a display of nature that will be forever etched in my memory. I stood motionless, not nearly ready to go on as my friend soon stopped to see what had startled me. He looked where I stared; there we were—both poised in time, momentarily capturing that which cannot be captured. I wonder if he remembers that day the way that I do…

All was soon to rest, less the waning sun—bent on a final gesture. Its last remnant of luster, by now—partially eclipsed, did thoroughly drench before me a somber patch of bare oak. Then at once their leafless silhouettes glistened with the radiance of brilliant amber, stoic and steadfast against a vermilion-stained sky. So still were the hands of time and even more evocative—the heartening horizon, I seemed then to have rekindled my verdant youth, thought long ago—lost to the ages.

In my time, I've often wondered on eternity, and how the day's truth differs from the nights'. Yet in the absence of resolve, there can be no truth more sound than that ambient landscape which has endured the fall of empires as well as sustained itself through the course of all times. Indeed, it was able to breathe life into a war torn will—just as mine; I'm left forever impressed by that moment. It was a brief window to the beginning of time, a mere peek at immortality.

As it continues, defying an ephemeral existence, so too will I persevere by the hand of its invincible virtue; that is, until I stay peacefully, outside of a way-worn mortal remain.

Those who seek everlasting existence must first live a life worth immortality.

When my time comes and I have exhausted the last of my life appropriately, I will tell those who mean to intervene with this natural course, to, "Let no man afflicted with society's ailing procedures molest my remains. Instead, let my ashes return to ashes—my dust to dust. Therefore, make ashes of me and let me alone to be dust in the everlasting wind." Everything that happens to me from here on, I want to be natural.

When we finally see that there are no such myths that are truly dreadful except in our minds, we will be free to live without burden; we will be free to live virtuously—with inner serenity.

I once pondered on this very matter during one of my stays in the hospital, when I was alone. It was one of the finest moments of clarity that I had known at that time in my life. That's why I remember it so well.

I was eight or nine stories high, looking out of the window—around one, two, or maybe three, in the morning. I noticed how the towering street lamps helped the stars light up the darkness. I could hear nothing but the soothing hiss of steam escaping beneath the vent that I leaned over to see the night's sky and a stray car here and there making its way home on Interstate 95. Other than that, the road was desolate.

A verse came to me as I realized that I was part of a larger movement that too struggled to find its way through uncertainty. It seems hauntingly ominous, but portrays a moment in time that I will never forget. It was how I felt right then when I thought about letting go of myths and embracing both life and death.

Alone in silence, on this, the longest night, I deeply consider all that will follow.

It is from here that I can see clearer than ever—far beyond tomorrow.

No longer forever can I deny the raven its rightful play; I know that time will come, so I must say farewell to each day's fading twilight.

Peculiar it is, how often will a tear trail a kiss; even more is, how in the midst of beauty, is sorrow.

To grasp once and for all—nothing is everlasting.

I feel this may be the moment to abandon—these myths of humankind; to see what others might never, that in the years to come—the dusk of man.

It is somehow beyond reach—beyond me.

All I can do is wonder, wait and let go—live, love and laugh; because my life is of time, and it too shall pass.

TO BE REBEL–YOUNG

An attitude that joins youth with maturity, rebellion with wisdom, bringing the best of both worlds together, is essential to living through life with health, confidence and vitality.

Unrest stirs the emerging generation. It has and always will; it is in our nature to distinguish ourselves from others, especially our elders. Young people are seldom satisfied with the way things have been, and wield their discontent in many directions of life. Their spirits are fresh and starving for meaning and purpose, not the kind that will suffocate them in time, but another manner of meaning that is much more sustaining. They long for a purpose that will nourish their spirits. They hear all the talk of freedom but see a society chained to the past. We notice their restlessness without a true understanding of its cause. We watch as they desperately free themselves of this past without responsibility—a sense of duty that must go hand in hand with liberation. We forget that they are the latest evolution in our revolutionary quest for independence and deliverance from conflict. To see them fail is ultimately, to see ourselves fail.

How we interpret youthful rebellion is our perception of their unwillingness to 'sit still' and conform to our ways, whatever that may be. But haven't we done the same? Aren't our ways simply of those before us? What is truly of our time that we bring to them beside the handed-down decadence from our previous generations? Is there anything original and exciting for them that would make them genuinely feel as if they were truly a part of something, that would make them feel like they were actually alive and not just living in the great eclipsing shadow of humanity? They need a new way…we all need a new way.

They do sense this new way, but they are not quite sure how to get there or even where to start. They know that it exists, which is just enough for them to hold onto. It is a very fragile hope. It depends so much on understanding and contribution from the rest of us. I wonder if we have enough love in our hearts to believe in them, to invest ourselves in their future, which is, in a way, our future?

Whether time or we, as their example—will ultimately smother this creativity, this extraordinary anticipation for life, which they possess, is what we must ask ourselves. It would be a great tragedy to desecrate such promise and hope against the impenetrable wall of our misunderstanding, or worse—our indifference.

Look into their eyes; you will see that there is a glorious vitality in them that was once ours as well. It hasn't left us but has only retreated within the deep recess of our spirit. Nothing is lost until we are gone; all can be revived, all can be rejuvenated.

When the next generation looks to us for the truth in life, will we give it to them, or only its shadow? And when they embrace it—and there is no substance, they will once again be without a way. The youth is not sure how they feel or why they are dissatisfied; all they know is that what they live is not enough, not anymore. We could learn a lot from their energy, daringness, and defiance. In fact, we should adopt their dissatisfaction with the course society has taken. We must be aware that the only thing separating the youth from the adult is a state of mind. Change your perspective and you'll change everything.

Wasn't there a time, maybe not so long ago, when you too wanted to feel like you were alive? When you too felt this same vibrant energy course through your veins, as you searched bravely for meaning and purpose in a world intent on smothering that breakaway spirit? You were like them—poised to change, and ready for anything. It felt good to be so bold—so imposing. This feeling is still with you. It waits within to emerge; it wants very much to spread its wings once again and brush off the dust of tradition.

The last generation felt it deeply, but unfortunately, squandered this energy. I know this, because I was able to see what took place on the television. I was a youthful boy then, yet I knew that something momentous was upon us. There was an attention to the news in my family unlike any other time. I could see that my parents were drawn to the events as they unfolded. To see so many gather with a common cause and attitude was encouraging. I may have been young, but I felt the magnitude of what I was witnessing take on its own life. It was at the time when our best had set foot on the moon. But for some reason, this event touched a deeper vein of our consciousness.

Nearly 500,000 of our youth eagerly gathered on the hills of Woodstock in the late sixties to "express themselves." It was a chance to stimulate change. Some could see that they were poised to do something remarkably original. The world waited—watching—secretly desiring to be there, desperately wanting to see something special come of it. So much was possible then, but what instead was the result? How was that energy spent? Who benefited by this? Was there an effort to broaden this energy to others in productive ways? Did they get together to discuss how they could make a difference in their culture? Or did they liberate themselves without this responsibility in a selfish, childish, portrayal of rebellion that appeared to many to look more like disobedience than a legitimate protest against corruption of the human spirit.

In the end, it came down to a self-serving display of misdirection. The news coverage had shown the progressive deterioration of order and unity to that of a disbanded mob of indulgence. That's what ultimately made the difference between causing a lasting change and stirring the muddy waters of monotony. It was, first of all, without direction—an aimless energy.

Those were tumultuous times and our country sought a different course. This would've been the start of a great ripple effect, indeed. That never happened. What reflected off the television screens in millions of homes became a spectacle of self-gratification. These beautiful people filled with aspirations and discontent, diffused their energy, abandoning it along the hills they gathered on, alongside the scattered debris left by their presence.

Instead of outwardly altering the world through passive influence, they took the easy way out, and in its place—altered their state of mind; many, with drugs and alcohol. So, in effect, they retreated from this world stage.

They had their chance and let it slip away, and ultimately got swallowed up by conformity. The remnants of that time are now but mere fragments of wonder, roaming nomadically throughout the participant's thoughts and forgotten dreams that once were, and for some, may never be again. They have fused well into society and many are successful in life.

The world has not changed. It still waits. But the rising hope of the world's peering eyes—still exists today. It has not gone away. It still remembers what was possible on those rolling hills of Woodstock, when war was in the air and blood was being spilled onto a distant land.

What's different now? Are the youth of today the very ones who can bring us back to feeling alive again? Will we join them this time? Can our spirits be redeemed, or are we traveling with too many burdens and responsibilities that we really don't need in our lives, both physically and emotionally? Have we slowly lost ourselves, and in doing so, followed the crowd, thinking it knew the way?

We must think about this deeply and not so easily dismiss it. Where do we often find feelings of such great passion and creativeness? Usually when we're forging a new way from the old, and when we stray from the familiar to the unknown. That's when our curiosity is heightened, as well as all of our senses. We feel that excitement welling up from within, like a great surge. We're not sure what's to come, but we can hardly wait.

Does the thought of adventure captivate you? Where do we find it today in our lives?

What place does it have in our spirit, if any? You might wonder what significance this has on health and disease. I say that when we're pursuing the best things in life, the noblest aspects of living with truth, our health observes that direction. It senses this confidence of being clear, deliberate and true. We are stimulated through and through. Every cell in our bodies is being nourished with meaning and purpose.

These are the moments in history that become opportunities to inspire, hope, bond, create change, and show who we are and what we are capable of. Anticipation of unity between people brings all these notions to life's table. This optimistic energy encourages and heals.

I'm not a young man anymore, although I try my best to stay fit. But I will tell you that my spirit is vigorous. I am aligned with the new generation. I'm right by their side, more than willing to let their active hope inspire me. I'm joining in the task of setting a new course that is full of life and beauty. The way lies just ahead of me. I know that I'm near where I should be because the genial sun is bright, lenient, and gentle on my face, like that of early morning or late afternoon. It forgives all that I've been through without judging me. I rely on its warmth. I let it drench my senses with its healing energy. It does just that. There are no strings attached to this gesture—no hidden agenda. That's the way it should be—ever renewing.

If ever I find myself unsure of the future or caught somewhere in the past, I have only to look to the skies to feel calm once again and to know where I am. I know that I'm a part of this immense and awesome timeless beauty, no matter what the past has done to me or what the future holds. I'm here right now—and I can see the sky.

I am aware now that I exist beyond the past, among the new generation, because I am open to their vision and welcome their discontent.

So when you think on such things as time and its effect on your life, remember to never fear the future or regret the past, but more than anything else, embrace the vitality and truth of the living moment. That's where you will find your true self; it is there that you will finally know God.

The elders bring wisdom, without which we would all be fated to repeat mistakes made in the past. So listen to them and bring them with you because in them survives—even if near death—a fervent child like wonder of what could possibly be. There is a side of everyone that is hopeful, no matter the age. Favor that side—give it care and attention.

Living rebel-young is understanding the importance of not accepting set ways of beliefs without seeking the truth and validity of these convictions. When there is attention to the moment and one is fully aware, there is a need to continually reevaluate thoughts, beliefs, and perceptions.

In this way, your thoughts will always be authentic, your beliefs will be true, and your perceptions will be clear. This will leave you with the vitality of youth.

Truth of the moment is as alive as any living thing in this world. If ever you should you lose your way in life, you will never find yourself by living in the past. You will only find remnants of what you were at one time; remnants of what the world was at one time. The truth of that moment is now subject to many interpretations, and with that confusion comes fear, doubt and anxiety.

The mind must be young at heart, but have wisdom guiding it. It should be venturous, creative, adaptable, aware, confident, quiet, undistracted, and with unusual sensitivity. A mind rebel-young should react not out of routine, but from curiosity. When one is living with an attitude that is rebel-young, one's mind is balanced. The creative mind is governing the inherent mind, and the human spirit is centered between, influencing the transactions in a continuous flow of energies. There is no conflict within or without, only understanding; and that understanding breeds a kind of confidence that is sustaining.

Striving to be rebel-young could not be more relevant to overcoming cancer or any other great adversity, whether it be any physical disease or an emotional imbalance. To be rebel-young is an attitude bolstered by the creative mind. It is a declaration of independence from fear and doubt. This is the very essence of self-empowerment. To be unaffected by distractions from the truth, to be uncompromising when challenged, to be steady in the face of uncertainty; all are qualities of living rebel-young.

We all lose when truth is sacrificed for denial. We end up imitating our way through life, and using our past as a symbolic crutch. This is exactly how the past survives death and is able to influence our thoughts and actions. Nothing new can emerge because it is overshadowed, and then we wonder why we feel lifeless and old before our time.

When I was young, I was well on my way to imitation. I began to fear what others feared. I doubted myself and what was possible. I discovered nothing but was shown everything.

Before I knew what this could do to me, it was already too late, and life's cold, unforgiving reality had found me.

Years before the accident, with my friend Dean, a seed of fear slipped into my mind, a fear of dying or of losing someone I loved. This fear of death stayed in my thoughts on and off throughout my adolescence. I had no sense of how to spend this fear—how to see through it, and understand its place in my life. I gave strength to an emotion far beyond its purpose. It was able to consume me, many times waking me up late at night. It lurked in the shadows of my mind, smothering the good thoughts that one should always enjoy when growing up.

I never let anyone know that I felt this way about things because I was strong-willed and felt that I had to work it out myself. I believed that living with conflict in the background of my thoughts was good enough to get by. I was wrong. It tainted every thought it touched. It had to be resolved in some way. For me, it was the hard way.

Veer well off the beaten path to find the true treasures in life. In your heart you know what they are. Stay fresh throughout life's trials and tribulations, and never blink when death attempts a stare down. Realize that the greatest strength lies in one's ability to adapt.

Never submit the creative mind to the inherent mind; this is an inward conformity. To truly be rebel-young is to resist the intimidation of the inherent mind; it is to remain steady on course with the creative mind at the helm—aware with attention to the moment. To be rebel-young is to be fearless at any age or in any condition. To be rebellious in this way is a revolutionary evolution of the mind. No matter what our age, it's never too late to feel young.

MOVEMENT AND
PROPER PROVISIONS

In staying with the theme of this book, which is maintaining balance throughout the body, mind and spirit for desired health, I cannot overlook the importance of adequate nutrition and keeping the body fit; it's always been a priority of mine. From the first time I learned of my cancer I knew that I needed to eat responsibly— even more so. I was already in good physical condition from years of strenuous activity. Discipline came natural to me because of this. Right away I started to look for the most nutritious foods that I could add to my daily intake.

There are many foods that are good for you and great tasting as well. True hunger and undistorted taste buds will lead you to the best foods for yourself, according to your individual needs. We have natural cravings that tell us what to eat, when to eat, and how much to eat, but we don't always listen to this intelligence within ourselves. And with the many influences around us, it is easy to dull this ability. Our internal influence can lapse from disregard. We must be responsible. There is no better time to follow your natural instinct than when you are not healthy. You will find that the body knows what it needs to heal itself, but you must be aware, you must give it attention. As it turns out, I did the right thing—I listened.

When I am exposed to the personal eating habits of my friends and extended family members, I notice how different mine are— compared to some. I see this even more with complete strangers who hadn't the influence of the way I lived, close to them. My family and friends watched my careful adherence to sound living. They saw how this helped me through my ordeal.

I respect every tradition and culture; each has a legitimate history of sustenance. The difference I'm talking about has little to do with this. It has to do with disregard. If it ain't broke, it's last on the list. If it ain't squeakin', it ain't getting oiled. This may be a crude description of some attitudes I've run across, but I think it's fair to say that many of us treat our health the way we treat our cars—that is, when something goes wrong, then it's time to do something about it.

The body is extremely tolerant and will go years enduring this neglect, but it will break down. The consequences of ignoring the needs of the body will manifest in the form of disease and vulnerability to infection.

First of all, let's talk about cancer and nourishment. Cancer's relation to nutrition is multi-dynamic. In this respect, we eat to feed the body and nourish the vital cells composing the immune system, which contains the all-important fighter cells. Within our white blood cells awaits an army of lymphocytes. To simplify, there is the B-lymphocyte and the T-lymphocyte, along with macrophages, which clean up and remove the cancer cells after they've been attacked and destroyed by the B&T lymphocytes. These cells are naturally influenced and persuaded by nutrition, right emotions, and the human spirit. They are very much alive and responsive to the direction of the whole body, mind and spirit. There is a striving for order, even at the cellular level. Within each living cell is a reflection of the greater organism in its entirety. It stands to reason that, within the very cell itself, exists the natural instinct to survive. We can properly nourish these cells, but without direction from the mind and the human spirit, without our emotions in check and steady, these fighter cells may still fail us.

On the other hand, we may be very steady with our emotions, but neglect to feed the cells with the essential nutrients for health, and in this way they may fail us as well.

I've heard prominent professionals and well experienced lay people declare the importance of a healthy diet. Some even take the position that diet alone can prevent, or cure even, cancer. Unfortunately, I do not hold this opinion. It is a partial truth that might bring a serious disappointment if solely adhered to on its own merit. To completely rely on nutrition as the answer, without maintaining balance concerning the whole body, would be like taking a car in for service and having the oil changed on schedule, but ignoring the brake fluid, spark plugs, transmission fluid, air filter, and tire pressure. Every working mechanism contributes to the integrity of the whole. Each needs attention. All serve to keep the car performing at optimal levels.

The body is similar. The same principles apply. Every part of it needs care and attention. There must be balance for there to be health. That is why this approach has not been universally accepted by the medical establishment. Health is much more dynamic than just what we eat. Proper nutrition followed moderately, with discipline, in its respective place, has the potential to prevent, even heal, as long as the balance in the body of all other relating entities is upheld.

What usually happens is that when the body falls ill, there is a systematic breakdown within the living system which might or might not involve the nutrition element only. When the body is compromised from improper nutrition, an array of diseases can surface that would manifest through these deficiencies, or indulgences in the various vices, such as over-exposure to the elements.

If we were to follow an excellent nutrition plan for a long period of time, prevention of disease would be greatly enhanced, but to get someone out of an acute situation, such as cancer or any life threatening disease where death is probable, diet alone would not be an adequate or responsible path of treatment in itself. This is why doctors will only advise eating soundly as a contributing factor to more conventionally accepted treatments. I certainly concur with this practice. It only makes sense. I cannot overstate the fact that there needs to be a dynamic approach to wellness. By all means, eat the best foods that you can—organic if possible, as close to fresh and in their natural state as you can find them. But remember, equal attention must be given to other requirements that keep the body optimal. There is a time and a place to rebel against conventional wisdom and also a time to exercise prudence, respect and observance to such. Hopefully, each one of you will know the difference, and therefore make sound judgments, after considering every aspect of your condition. No one ever said this was going to be easy, but I'm saying it's doable.

With that said, knowing now what role nutrition plays in the theater of illness, at least where there is an immediate danger, we can understand that when it comes to cancer and its unpredictability, nutrition becomes a requisite for nourishing the body, while it fends off the progression of disease. In this way, diet is crucial to an overall protection carried out by the internal relating systems of defense, and the creative-inherent mind—fully influenced by the human spirit. I have reduced my plan to a simple method so as to not complicate my life any more than it has been. This has worked well for me. I eat when I am hungry and drink when I'm thirsty. I don't mind what others say about this, I listen to my body when it speaks. In this way do I know when the body is ready for nutrition, and in need of water. I say water because, of all my convictions, none is held more adamantly than the belief that we should consume predominantly water as our hydrating source. There is no debate; clean water is life-giving and essential in its natural state.

The thing to pay attention to when one listens to the body is the first hunger pangs. You'll notice at first that the initial hunger pangs feel right. They give a good sensation that feels appropriate. This is the time to eat; not hour's later but right then. The problem arises when people ignore this initial signal and wait till it hits again and again, until it becomes a painful hunger pang and doesn't feel right anymore. At this point, after ignoring these natural signals, the body gets the wrong message and thinks that it is starving. And by this inner perception, it goes into a starvation mode. This is a condition where the body begins to use its own muscle for protein and precious glucose stores for energy, which is why we feel so strange and irritable after we've neglected these initial signs. In the same way does the body draw water from its lesser tissues to hydrate the organs which are more important to the living system; this happens when thirst has been disregarded as well. There's no thought process here, it's instinctive. This is why it's vital to act immediately when the subtle hunger pangs and thirst first come to you. There is a window of opportunity for the individual to be responsible rather than having to adhere to a regimen based on timeline, which is unnatural and confining. I mean, why eat if there's no hunger? Why drink if one is not thirsty?

Forget all the scare tactics and concerns; look at it simply. To feel hungry is healthy. It is a sign of right condition. Just listen to the signs when they come. Be sensitive to the body's needs. Act on them immediately. The body has a remarkable intelligence. But we do have choice. This separates us from this intelligence. We must bridge this barrier by choosing to listen to our body when it signals. It is the individual's responsibility to do the right thing, which is to eat when hungry and drink when thirsty.

After time, you will be in tune with your body's needs and your body will have a balance and confidence in you—as its master. Having said this, it is another thing completely to have extenuating circumstances that change the natural state of requirements in the individual. For instance, during cancer treatments, one may not be hungry for unnatural reasons; such as when experiencing the side effects of chemotherapy or radiation. In this case the rules have changed. Now, one is forced to eat without being hungry, and drink without being thirsty.

When something out of the ordinary alters the natural state of the individual, one must adapt and change methods accordingly. The many health conditions afflicting people have caused the individual to have unnatural requirements placed upon him or her, making it very difficult to listen to the body, because the body at this point is out of balance, and by this—stressed. This is why I speak generally when I say that one should be able to listen to the messages given by the body. In a diseased state, the body is somewhat, but not totally, incapable of speaking for itself; and until it has returned to its natural state, the individual should adjust his method of nutrition with this in mind.

For example, if there is a weight deficit due to illness or therapies, then one must eat more to compensate for this.

When it comes to how much the individual should eat at one time, I have thoughts on this as well. Leave the table when you can eat a little more; that is, when you're not quite full. This is a good rule of thumb. It allows the body to digest food easier and prevents the body from being overburdened with distributing surplus calories. It also leaves the body the energy to perform other necessary actions that are ongoing, especially when one is ill. One can always eat again in increments, which to me is the desired method of eating. Small meals spaced throughout the day will keep one alert and mildly hungry with the body's engine always in a revved-up condition.

Food should be in its closest natural state as possible. Try to consume it with most of its nutrients still intact. This means, don't overcook food in any way—whether in steaming, broiling, sautéing, and so on. Notice I didn't mention frying; enough said. I like my crispy food too, but all in moderation. While we're talking about taboos, table salt is one of the biggest for me. If anything, I prefer an occasional sprinkle of the mineral rich higher-end sea salts. Other than this, stay away from too much salt. Hydrogenated oils of any kind are off limits as well; they are deadly. Refined sugars, bleached flours, and denatured grains eaten in excess are empty, valueless calories.

Generally, try to make the times that you eat opportunities to nourish, not simply satisfy the senses. Use your calories wisely by getting the most nutrients from your food. Also, make eating a pleasurable thing by sitting down and taking the time to enjoy what you consume. Try not to shove it down your throat in a hurry, because it will make your digestion—work that much harder. Start digestion first in the mouth, when chewing your food well. This is sound advice. I'll never forget the eastern philosophy when it comes to thoughts on eating. One proverb goes a long way: *"Drink your food and chew your liquid."* I couldn't have said it better.

When I think about the many years of practice and play that I participated in through my adolescence, during the cruel heat of the late summer, and after a long day at school, where everyone else could go home but we, (my teammates and I) stayed till the evening, practicing and practicing—I was constantly in motion. My movements were graceful and appropriate for my age; my lungs, strong and seldom winded. My timing and reflexes were keen and spot on. My footsteps were swift and nimble. This came natural to me. It wasn't a chore. It felt normal because it was a part of my schedule. It was all I knew.

Life moves with intention, direction, and most importantly, out of necessity. From the slow growth of a seed into a tree, from within a single honeycomb bursts a bee—life propels. In the interval, it rests and reserves, only for the energy to once again vitally stir. We are no different. We must see the truth in balancing these implementations, so that no one course is overextended. As we all know very well, too much of anything can be counterproductive. Overeating can excessively burden digestion, further taxing the organs responsible for the process of assimilation, and cause the body to store unneeded calories in the way of fat. Too much rest can make one lethargic, and begin the progression of muscular atrophy, allowing the sediments of infection to settle and take hold. Closer to the point, too much exercise prevents the body from repairing itself through rest and recovery. Each and every scenario can eventually stress the living system into illness, which is really caused by an imbalance somewhere along the way; evidence of moderation turned to excessiveness. This will eventually lead to a systemic breakdown. These are the physical characteristics of inconsistency.

Shortly after I returned home from the hospital following a stay in isolation for several weeks, with my body having been greatly traumatized, I began to realize how weak I'd been rendered from the effects of immobility, infection and sleep deprivation. The continuing pain and lack of caloric intake—outside of a maintenance of IV fluids, which is simply glucose and not by any means an elixir capable of sustenance for any extended period of time—prevented me from motion. Every muscle of mine sagged; standing up, even briefly, brought dizziness and a feeling of fatigue. My weight had plummeted from 150 to 107 lbs. I was literally skin and bones. There was hardly a semblance of my former self in the mirror. I could only remember what I once looked like. Every cell in my body remembered too— what I used to be. All they needed was to be nudged and influenced in some way.

Something else occurred to me during that pivotal point in my life, as if I didn't have enough to overcome. I realized that while I had honed my physical strength through my formative years, I had allowed my mind to atrophy from lack of use—lack of motion—if you will. I didn't realize then, that even the mind must move as much as any other part of the body. It must be observing, imagining and creating, ever again and again. Beliefs we hold must be occasionally reconsidered, whatever they may be. Thoughts we have should at times stimulate and inspire. What we've learned must be looked at deeply, with reason, logic and most importantly—our own opinion. The knowledge we hold within our mind must be exposed to the light of day and given a dose of fresh air from time to time. I consider these movements to be of a different kind, but no less vital.

We have to see how we're part of a whole living system in which most other living things move instinctively, where we have the luxury to decide whether we want to or not—and this is where choice is not negotiable—when living the higher laws. With this freedom of decision comes a certain responsibility to adhere to the principles of nature, which all fall under the rule of the higher laws; and these are divine—in that they are where creative intelligence exists in totality. Flowing through us is the mystery of intuition, natural instinct, creativity, and most of all, the force and will of the human spirit—all of which transcends the known into the unknown. When we are in that flow—in the zone, we see the best in us at work. It is then that we are living these higher laws appropriately.

The human body is remarkably resilient. It will certainly accommodate our vices and bend to our behaviors, but only for so long. It will obey our desires and stand up to our exploitations, even under prolonged conditions of such abuse and neglect. But if we do not listen to its needs, it will first show symptoms of pain and fatigue, and eventually give way to disease.

There must be great attention given to the care of the whole body, mind and spirit. Remember, spirituality is an ever-flowing vital energy, deserving the utmost respect. Attention to our behavior is another form of movement. Our relationship with others is a movement in itself; it is a movement of love, compassion, empathy, forgiveness, care, kindness, consideration, concern, sacrifice, and other such ways of the heart. These are the movements of grace and beauty; these are movements with meaning.

When we observe those around us, do we hear creativity in their words, or are they as stagnant and uninspiring as a sermon on the dreadful affects of straying from the herd, as a preacher might forewarn? Is their imagination as encompassing as a painter or poet; or have they fallen into habit, boredom and predictability? For I have seen, returning back into society from an extensive leave, that people are settling for so much less than what is their god-given right. I've noticed too, that our minds our heavily burdened with indifference, and we have lost a deep sense of appreciation for the most important things in life. We have forgotten what it is to yearn for something real and exciting, something that could possibly make our hearts beat strong and vibrantly—again, as when we were children and everything was new, innocent, and turned over for the first time. Isn't this all a movement of some kind? Doesn't habit, ritual, and routine, prevent this movement?

To see this is to realize that no matter what distraction we choose, whether of the mind or of the body, each is a vice that's relief is only temporary. We are still held within the confines of our social inheritance. Escape is not a movement; it is simply a distraction.

There must be a revolution of the spirit to indeed break free of our prisons that have been decorated with the ordinary. We must be ready to change, however uncertain and uncomfortable it may be to do so; simply because truth is in that next unknown. This is what it is to be with attention to the moment, which, in itself, is a graceful, poised, movement of the mind.

The body, mind and spirit, can be paralyzed by thoughts and emotions as well. Fear, despair, frustration, guilt, hatred, anger, jealousy, and similar feelings can be very detrimental to the creative movement which is essential to vitality and health, as is discussed in the chapter, *Emotions that Wither.*

To move gracefully, both in mind and in body—to have appropriate thoughts and deliberate right actions emanating from those thoughts—is to move with purpose. This will emulate confidence, the kind of confidence that will attract others; like a ripple beginning in the center, working its way out towards humanity. This is how we change the world, by slight eddying currents of evolving movements of the whole mind and body.

It is an essential part of life to move. So many aspects of survival rely on our ability to let in the life force around us and replenish our cells with life sustaining elements. By deliberate movements, we are also stimulating each cell in our bodies to release toxins; toxins that are by-products of cellular activity, and from continued ingestion of foreign contaminants. A body in motion gathers necessary nutrients from the bloodstream, inhales fresh oxygen through the lungs, and keeps every cell at attention and in concert with each other, at all times.

There are so many forms of motion that are good for us; it is suggested to explore the possibilities individually, according to one's preference. I would like to mention some that I believe are worth noting. To me, nothing compares to the practice of stretching. Its effects are miraculous, and everyone can participate. Continued stretching makes one limber in time, which is very healthy for the body. It elongates the muscles and sends the blood rushing through them. The idea here is to get as far away from stiffness as one is able to. There is no life in a stale, rigid, body *or* mind.

Walking is a favorite of mine because you receive all the benefits of movement without the trauma on the joints that say, running on a hard surface might cause. It is a great low-impact exercise; one you can perform socially as well. Take a walk on the shoreline as you listen to the waves crash beside you. This can be very soothing or invigorating, depending on your mood.

If you're near a lake or pond instead, you might rejoice at the serenity of the still water. It really doesn't matter what form of movement you prefer, so long as you are in motion.

As far as a movement of the mind, start to think creatively in ways you would have never thought before. Look at things from an entirely different perspective. Inquire into everything that intrigues you. Be curious. Think of ideas that might help others or yourself. Find the path to inspiration in what you love. Imagine acts of compassion throughout the day and then perform them, even little ones. Be spontaneous and surprise those around you. Try to shake things up a little. Stop putting off what you really want to do and find a way to do it; your spirit will appreciate the effort.

Reach out to others who might need you; you'll never know how much you're wanted until you try. What a feeling it would be to have someone, even a stranger, look you in the eye and smile with great appreciation for caring about them or taking the time to listen. How rare is that these days—to really listen? This is what strengthens the heart and spirit. This is the revolution I refer to, a revolution of perspective, of change—a revolution of motion!

EPILOGUE

All throughout our lives we will experience conflict and confidence, struggle and peace; many Goliaths will overshadow the way; states of mind existing within ourselves, realities of life around us. Some would even argue that we are defined by this disparity. What is important is how we handle the life cycles that challenge us personally, and the things we do about these imbalances in our world that test our resolve as a people. Perception and interpretation of what is in fact actual may very well be our greatest Goliath of all.

It can be a normal reaction to search outwardly for answers to why unfortunate things happen, because blame can sometimes be a tough pill to swallow—both individually and as a responsible race. In both cases, our true enemy remains human weakness, vanity, and a rooted fear of death, caused by a lack of understanding and awareness to the moment. All give way to our compulsions, taking us further from beauty, purity, the virtues, and vitality. Each and every sacrifice of principle or ethic for short term gain and immediate satisfaction strips yet another layer of armor from what ought to be our impenetrable will to live. A gradual, undetectable loss of heart begins the inevitable degradation of the human spirit, where at last its remaining embodiment withers, naked—abandoned by all gods, mysteries and freedoms.

I don't have to look too closely to see that I've been directly impressed upon by my continued defiance through the years; outwardly the signs of this are clearly there, right before me. I have scars and sutures decorating my body. My face is no longer smooth, but rough from disseminating shingles. My once muscular frame is unnaturally slender from wasting *and* from the direct effect of radiation. My veins are hard to see, and even harder to find when I require blood work—compliments of chemotherapy. My five o'clock shadow reveals more and more grey hairs replacing my naturally pitch-black ones. Some might say that wisdom replaces ignorance in such a way, that is, through hardship. I would tend to agree, unfortunately, not without some degree of forgoing a simple life. So, I've been shown, is the way of life.

Adversity calls upon our reserves like no other situation is ever able to. It's in these troubled times that you find out what's real and what isn't, about yourself, and about life.

At times, I was apprehensive, but not enough to be afraid. I was lost in the newness of my environment, yet I refrained from seeking direction. I respected life's impositions, but not nearly enough to yield to them. I went from reacting to life, to imposing my will on it; I had to.

Disease can be a runaway destructive force, but it is by no means senseless; this thought is an illusion, held up by misunderstanding. On the other hand, health is a much more vital energy than illness will ever be. The universe favors the living and its vitality. In other words, it tends towards order, and this is good news for us, because health is a balanced system working in harmony—working in order. However, there are constant anomalies present within this imperfect universe. To trick the mind into order, through turning away from what is actual, is a foolish endeavor. To seek security from what is actual takes one further from truth.

What I'm suggesting is not an easy road to take, we must remember, our greatest struggle will lend us our greatest strength. All else will degrade our spirit's ability to bond with the healing force.

There is an amazing capacity for the human being to be resilient in times of overwhelming adversity. We see this phenomenon in every facet of our existence, though at times it seems an esoteric notion that escapes the majority of people, which is not the case at all. The intelligence of survival rests solely upon the individual, to first understand the dynamic self and its relating entities, and when armed with this familiarity, realize its relation to nature and humanity in a balance of inner and outer entities.

This totality of awareness is the beginning of living responsibly in accordance with the higher laws of life. It is a new way of self-empowerment that has been long overdue. To center one's attention in this manner, when the world is distracting us on so many different strata, both subtly and openly, is not an easy thing to do. But if one sees the importance of what I have come to know as a result of living through cancer, that individual will be inspired to also create a new way.

This kind of inspiration is very contagious, and by extension, will eventually gain its own momentum. It is an influence pure and genuine.

I'm confident that the therapy of the future will involve vaccines of all types. What do vaccines do but stimulate the immune system into action?

So we are coming full circle in science and medicine, back to the most promising defense known to humanity. It is within each one of us already, at this very moment. We have the ability right here and now—to directly influence the immune system with our mind and spirit, through thoughts and actions. So why wait for science to confirm this potential? Do we have this time to spare, this luxury? Trust yourself, know yourself, motivate yourself in a way that gives you back control over your life—in reality, not simply in words, or with a sense of vagueness. There are legions of fighters out there living through adversity each and every day. We should look to them for their ability to not give in. They have an abundance of qualities to offer humanity, because they hold the key to life locked in their experience. If we are with enough sensitivity and attention, then maybe, just maybe, we will learn from their lives; and even from their deaths. That's right…I've seen how heroes live and die—I knew one.

Cancer will never define me. My defiance in the face of cancer will reflect who I really am.

Life has shown me many things, but most importantly, it has shown me that nothing is irretrievable. Life rejuvenates strength, the spirit, love, vitality, and above all things—innocence, of which without, none of the aforementioned could ever exist. Not the innocence of naiveté, nor the innocence of ignorance, but the pure innocent temperance of creativity and will.

We've asked two inescapable questions, consistently, throughout time: What is our purpose in life, and what is the meaning of us being here? I see it simply. A clear answer surfaces for those like me, who come so close to death. My purpose in life is to survive and help others survive with the same intensity. I gain meaning in life in this very endeavor.

From the moment we come into this world we are faced with our own Goliaths. Some will experience more profound challenges than others, simply because life is not fair. The presence of adversity is as natural as the change of seasons. Death is the ultimate Goliath, not to be slain or denied—but understood and held at bay. Defy death daily; defy it for a lifetime!

Just as there are many Goliaths in life, there are also potential Davids out there, who bleed the same vital blood as he bled, shed the same fearless tears as he once did, and breathe the courageous breath from the same air of the ages. Be that legendary David and defy your Goliath—gloriously! Endure all!

David Michael Como Jr.

IN THOUGHT
AND REMEMBRANCE

To my brothers—Louis and Tommy; thanks for always being there for me. I saw more attention than the both of you, though you never held it against me—never.

Willingly, in grateful debt to my stepfather; it's been a long road for you I'm sure, and knowing the man that you are, one you would gladly travel again—if necessary. Your commitment to our family is admirable and greatly respected. You alone made me aware of the need to volunteer and donate, through observing the way that you lived. I was watching. Thank you George

And to my father, who showed me more courage in thirty days than I have known from him in my lifetime. I wish you were here to read this book. I know that you would've been proud. I love you and you're missed often.

Dean, words will never be enough to express how having you ripped away from me, because of me, has affected me. I hope by now that you've forgiven me. I've just begun the task of forgiving myself.

Linda, I smile even now, some twenty-seven years later, because I remember everything we shared together. You were the one. Life offered me my true love long before I realized it, long before I could appreciate it, and for this...I lost you. You've haunted me like no other. Traces of you remain in my heart.